COME RIDE WITH ME

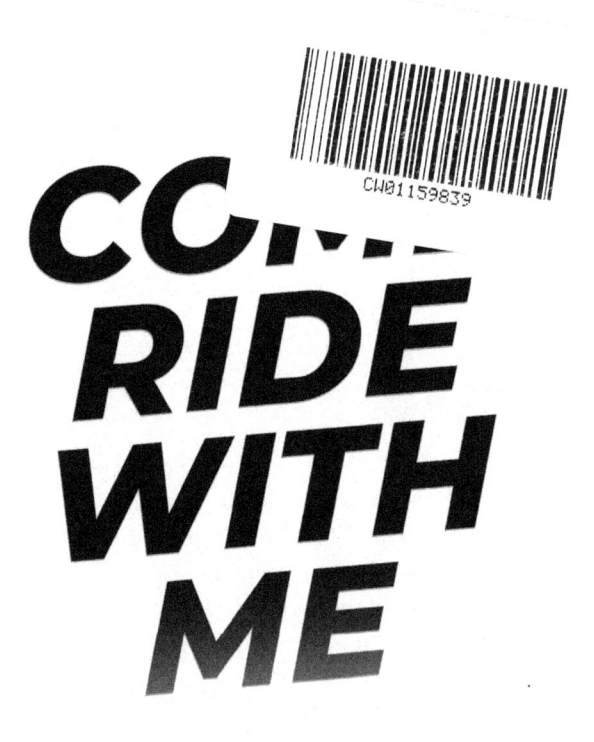

MEMOIRS OF A PARAMEDIC

STEVE KAWAMURA

Come Ride With Me
Copyright © 2023 by Steve Kawamura

All rights reserved. No part of this publication may be reproduced, distributed, or transmitted in any form or by any means, including photocopying, recording, or other electronic or mechanical methods, without the prior written permission of the author, except in the case of brief quotations embodied in critical reviews and certain other non-commercial uses permitted by copyright law.

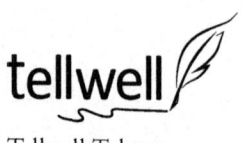

tellwell

Tellwell Talent
www.tellwell.ca

ISBN
978-0-2288-9460-5 (Hardcover)
978-0-2288-9459-9 (Paperback)
978-0-2288-9461-2 (eBook)

This book is dedicated to all the first responders who put on a uniform before work and willingly step into the unknown.

*Prepare for the worst, hope for the best.
Keep it simple if you can, and always look before you leap.
Advice to my paramedic students.*

TABLE OF CONTENTS

Wax On, Wax Off ix

Chapter 1	Bodily Fluids	1
Chapter 2	Motor Vehicle Collisions	10
Chapter 3	Paramedic Dilemmas	20
Chapter 4	The Mentally Ill	35
Chapter 5	Fire	46
Chapter 6	Unpalatable Places	58
Chapter 7	The COVID-19 Pandemic	68
Chapter 8	Remarkable People	87
Chapter 9	Frequent Flyers	100
Chapter 10	Shots Fired!	110
Chapter 11	Till Death Do Us Part	121
Chapter 12	Succumbing to Mental Illness	127
Chapter 13	The Obviously Dead	138
Chapter 14	The Paranormal	148
Chapter 15	That's Not in My Job Description!	157
Chapter 16	Trauma	168
Chapter 17	Lucky	177
Chapter 18	Saves	187

Epilogue 199

I would like to acknowledge all the wonderful people I have had the privilege to work with over the years. Not only my fellow paramedics, but hospital staff and allied first responders.

WAX ON, WAX OFF

Thanks for coming along for a ride in the ambulance. In 1986, I saw *The Karate Kid* on VHS, which ignited my first passion, karate. I competed all over the United States and Canada, earning many national and international championships.

As I approached the end of high school, I had to decide what I wanted to do with the rest of my life. I'm an action junkie, so an office job wasn't for me, but my GPA of 4.1 opened up a number of doors. My guidance counsellor was surprised when I applied for a co-op with the fire department. I told him this was what I wanted to do, but he strongly suggested I would be closing some doors by not attending university. I landed a co-op placement with Ancaster Fire and Emergency Service, the only fire service in Ontario to run an ambulance. When I found out I couldn't be a firefighter because I was colour blind, I shifted my focus to the medical calls.

I loved every minute of it.

Since the ambulance went to many of the same calls as the firefighters, we would all meet back at base after a call and discuss it in detail. What worked, what didn't, and what could work better. One day, a syncope (fainting) call went out that turned out to be a cardiac arrest. An advanced care paramedic, (those who possess a higher skill set than a primary paramedic and can administer different drugs) from another service attended with us. He was so confident and smooth, his hands moving quickly and with conviction. It wasn't only apparent to me; the firefighters noticed it too.

"I'm glad that guy showed up; he's good," one of the firefighters said with a nod.

Barely eighteen years old, I resolved to become a paramedic who earned the respect of allied emergency services. So, I made it my second passion. It would take many sleepless nights and years of effort to reach that goal. I kept notes on those calls and continuously learned valuable lessons, especially from the ones where I made mistakes. It helped me become a better paramedic.

Eventually, I had so much material that I decided to write about it. This book is a compilation of over twenty years of the most notable calls that I have had the privilege to attend. I cannot take credit for anything without mentioning how essential my work partners and the allied first responders are. My family and friends also supported me through the hard times.

I pull no punches and narrate the calls as meticulously as I can remember. This book is not for the faint of heart, and there are realities I faced on the streets of Hamilton that may make some readers uncomfortable.

Let me pause here to spend a minute on my hometown, Hamilton, Ontario. It is a unique city located at the head of Lake Ontario. With a population of about 535,000, it is tremendously diverse. In a matter of a thirty-minute drive you can go from farmland to inner city, to wine country. The Niagara Escarpment separates the lower city from what Hamiltonians call "The Mountain." The natural wonder provides the platform for many of its' over one hundred waterfalls. Imports and exports flow through the harbour, and the city was once home to a prosperous steel industry. Though the steel mills still run, they operate at a fraction of what they did in the 1980s, but many other interests prosper here.

The film industry has a strong presence in this city. *The Handmaid's Tale*, *The Incredible Hulk* and *X-Men* are just a few titles. McMaster University hosts one of the most prominent medical schools in Canada. The Ti-Cats keep the CFL fans here occupied, while artists of all kinds display and sell their work in many of the local art stores in the downtown core. These are just some of the things that are attractions to the area.

The urban core is one of the most poverty-stricken areas in Canada, so it provides a dynamic work environment for a paramedic. I would never say I've seen it all, but Hamilton has provided me a chance to say I've seen enough.

Some details have been changed to protect confidential sources, and I secured permission to tell the stories of the individuals named. At the end of each chapter, I have a song selection that themes it. Music has always been an important healer in my life.

Chapter 1

Bodily Fluids

The human body is a masterpiece of biological machinery. How it accomplishes daily tasks is nothing short of miraculous. But like any well-oiled machine, it requires fluids to do this—many different types of fluids.

Paramedics are exposed to all kinds: saliva, amniotic sac fluid, blood, cerebrospinal fluid, bone marrow, urine and diarrhea are just a few. During my career, I have been covered in many of them. To protect myself, I always have my personal protective equipment (PPE) ready at hand. This includes gloves, gowns, a face shield, safety glasses and isolation suits for the over-the-top exposures.

The COVID-19 pandemic shone a spotlight on PPE. For the first time in human history, the general public would be required to don it in most places. We wore masks on every call from the day the pandemic was declared. I thought about the twenty years I was in the patient compartment of the ambulance without a mask and how many sick patients were coughing in an enclosed space. Suddenly, a mask wasn't a bad idea. Since it is so easy to get covered in bodily fluids, I welcomed the idea with open arms. As you'll see, I should have had more PPE on in some of the following circumstances …

Season: Fall
Time: 1500hrs
Weather: Warm, 15°C
Area Demographic: Senior's apartments
Dispatch Info: Unresponsive 85yo female

I found the patient, a petite, elderly woman, on the bathroom floor of the apartment. I estimated her to be just over four feet and maybe one hundred pounds. I tried to wake her but could not. She only moaned to me, and her blood pressure was extremely low. I started an IV and got her blood pressure up. Within a few minutes, she woke up and started talking to us. She told us that she was trying to have a bowel movement when she passed out. She was a sweet woman who possessed the politeness and manners I enjoy in the elderly. Passing out on the toilet this way is actually quite common. Bearing down too hard to have a bowel movement can cause a rapid drop in blood pressure and heart rate, so the person passes out.

After we secured the patient on the stretcher, she made an urgent request to return to the toilet and finish the job she started. I hastily declined her request for fear that her blood pressure might drop, causing her to pass out again. This was a big mistake.

During transport to the hospital, the woman suddenly blurts out, "I'm sorry—it's gonna be bad!"

Seconds later, I gagged and put on a mask because the stench made me want to vomit. It smelled like something died inside her a year ago and was finally making its way out. A few moments later, I heard what sounded like molasses hitting the ambulance floor and I saw a steady flow of feces the consistency and colour of half-melted chocolate ice cream coming off the foot end of the stretcher. It sure didn't smell like ice cream. The liquid magma of feces oozed towards me at an alarming rate. I remembered my partner had his personal belongings on the floor, so I frantically threw his things from the back into the front of the ambulance. He asked me if he should step on the accelerator to get us there faster, but I pleaded with him not to as the extra speed may cause the lake of excrement to splash onto me.

Eventually, we got to the hospital and took the patient out of the ambulance. The puddle of waste was over a metre and a half in diameter, and we dragged the stretcher wheels right through it, leaving skid marks on the pavement. I felt bad for the hospital orderlies, so I cleaned it up. My soon-to-be wife also got to share in the moment when I sent her a pic of the floor of the ambulance with the text, "I'm gonna be late."

Season: Fall
Time: 1330hrs
Weather: Cold, windy, 8°C
Area Demographic: Long-term care facility
Dispatch Info: 55yo male, leg wound

Dispatch told us that the patient was potentially over 350 pounds and we might need the bariatric stretcher, an automatic stretcher capable of carrying up to one thousand pounds. There was only one and the policy stated we had to make patient contact first to call for it. Then a separate crew had to drive to the base and pick up that special ambulance, which creates a delay in transporting the patient.

Upon patient contact my eyes widened. This man was enormous—minimum 450 pounds. When paramedics come across a patient this big, we automatically think of back injuries. During the years before automatic stretchers, I would see at least one medic a year go down with a career-ending injury that would impact them for the rest of their life. Back and shoulders were the most common areas that were affected. I've spent time recovering from both. This happened less frequently when we got the automatic stretchers. It always took effort to hide my facial expressions when I came into visual contact with a bariatric patient because I associated them with severe injury.

We radioed dispatch for the bariatric stretcher, and they informed us it would take a while because we were short a couple of trucks. With that, we concentrated on the situation at hand. The patient said he struck his calf on the edge of the bed and thought nothing of it. There was a small hematoma (blood sac) that had tripled in size since the incident an hour ago. While waiting for the bariatric stretcher to arrive, I drew a circle around the hematoma with my pen. I watched it grow exponentially before my eyes. When the bariatric stretcher finally came forty-five minutes later, the hematoma had grown to the size of a ripe spaghetti squash. The skin had been stretched thin like a balloon and could burst at any second.

We needed six people to move the patient over to the stretcher. We assigned one nurse to guide that leg over. During the movement I could see the hematoma moving, and despite our best effort, it burst like a water balloon exploding! Blood splashed all over my gloved hands and legs, and I immediately put a pressure dressing on the wound to stop the bleeding. My partner got more dressings, applied pressure and got the bleeding under control.

The blood had gotten inside my gloves and covered my palms. Both my legs had blood stains on the skin that soaked through my uniform. The nurses immediately informed me that the patient was on a cytotoxic drug, which meant I'd been potentially exposed to radiation, but I didn't have time to deal with this at the moment.

We hastily transported the patient to the hospital. After we dropped the patient off, I called my supervisor and got some time to clean up. We looked up the drug and discovered it was only dangerous if swallowed. It always amazed me we have drugs that are given routinely that are considered a hazard.

When I followed up on the patient, I found out he had gone into hypovolemic shock and ended up in ICU for a couple of weeks. Eventually, he made it back to the nursing home.

Season: Summer
Time: 0800hrs
Weather: Hot, hazy, humid, 35°C
Area Demographic: Apartment, urban core
Dispatch Info: Woman in labour, language barrier

This call was dispatched to us as a non-emergency call, so I could not drive with my lights and sirens on. Dispatch told us that there was a language barrier, so information was scattered at best. What they could decipher was that this was the woman's third pregnancy. Well, it didn't take a doctor to figure out that this was an emergency, so I hounded dispatch to change the status so I could turn on the lights and step on the gas.

After a few minutes we were finally upgraded to emergency status and we arrived at the scene. A short, thin man who spoke little English met us in the lobby of the apartment buildings. His skin was dark black and he was dressed in long bright colourful robes. All he could say was hello, and he kept nodding at the questions I asked. He smiled politely and walked with a cane.

The man sauntered up to the apartment where ten people were standing around a young woman that I estimated to be in her twenties who was curled up in a ball on the floor. The people were all dressed in the robes

I mentioned earlier and had very dark skin. I wasn't sure where they were from due to the language barrier. There was no look of concern on their faces or sense of urgency in their body language. The patient was stoic and only quietly whimpered.

The baby bump on her abdomen was enormous, so I quickly ushered her onto the stretcher. I took a family member to help with what little translation would happen. I was always patient and courteous when dealing with non-English speaking families. It is so common here that you get used to it. I keep in the back of my mind that my family didn't speak English when they came here over three generations ago.

Through a game of charades and makeshift sign language, I deciphered this was the woman's third pregnancy. Her contractions may have started the previous night, and her water may have broken already. I gestured to her to tell me when she thought the baby was coming and she nodded.

On route, she grabbed my hand, looked me in the eye and screamed—a universal sign for "This baby is coming now!" Despite my fifteen years of experience, I had never delivered a baby. She was grabbing my hand so tightly I had trouble pulling away. Without hurting her, I wriggled free and opened the obstetrics kit for the first time in my career. I placed a pad underneath the patient's buttocks.

WHOOOOSH!

A gush of amniotic fluid hit me from my chest to my knees! Well, now I knew for sure that her water didn't break last night. We rushed to the hospital, and the baby's head was visible as we were in the elevator to the obstetrics floor. We made it to the labour and delivery room. She delivered a healthy baby boy seconds after we transferred her off of the stretcher. The cries of a healthy newborn baby brought a sense of inner warmth and a smile to my face.

I would have stayed and congratulated the family, but I was desperate to change clothes. The hospital lent me a set of greens, and let me use their change room. I had a summer uniform golf shirt that had to be pulled over your head. They had just come out and were great in the heat of the summer. I made several attempts to pull it over my head without it touching my face, but it seemed impossible and the smell was making me nauseated. So, like the Incredible Hulk when he's angry, I just ripped it in two and threw it in the biohazardous waste bin at the hospital. Now, I dreaded taking off my pants. I didn't know what areas were wet on my underwear but breathed a big sigh of relief when I saw that my groin area was bone dry. Just my hip was soaked with the amniotic fluid. *Phew!*

On the next call …

I got so used to being covered in every fluid imaginable that it eventually translated to my personal life. I would change a baby and get poop all over my hands or clothes or help someone who was bleeding all over the place. Never bothered me.

But the one thing I still don't like is vomit.

Like many of us in our early twenties, I was exposed to vomit during my bar-hopping days. Those times are long gone, but I'm occasionally reminded of it on a Friday night shift when the bars close. I still gag a little when I find out what my patient has tried to soak up the alcohol with.

Chapter song selection:
"Party Til You Puke" by Andrew W. K.

Chapter 2

Motor Vehicle Collisions

When two vehicles collide at high speed, you never know what is going to happen. The energy that is created is compounded, causing massive damage to the vehicles and their occupants. Sometimes people walk away from collisions that look like a battle between two scrap heaps. Sometimes there are fatalities where the damage seems minimal.

Either way, motor vehicle collisions are a crossroads for first responders—an arena where we come together in a coordinated effort to help patients. The police provide scene safety and investigative efforts. The fire department are masters of extrication. Then there is us, overlords of patient care. The outcome of the patient relies on all first responders performing well together and individually. To the average bystander, it looks like anarchy. But to us, it is organized chaos at its finest.

COME RIDE WITH ME

Season: Fall
Time: 0230hrs
Weather: Cool, 10°C
Area Demographic: 100km/h highway
Dispatch Info: Car vs. transport truck

My partner and I were going back to base and talking about calls. She told me that she did a call on this exact highway for a car going the wrong way on the road at around this time of night. At that exact moment, a car travelling in the opposite direction flashed its high beams at us. We didn't know why at the time, but we would soon find out.

Dispatch called to tell us there was a car versus transport truck just ahead of us. We looked at each other in shock. What a coincidence!

Within a few minutes, we were on-scene. The first thing I noticed was a transport truck with its front end totally smashed in. I found out later the vehicle had been walloped with such force that the engine was knocked off its mount. The driver was outside talking to a firefighter and seemed okay. His nonchalant body language suggested he was not injured. My partner went to talk to him anyway to confirm our look test while I rushed to the other vehicle.

It was a pickup truck, and the whole front cab had been squished like an accordion. The bumper and front wheel were underneath the driver's side door, and the windshield had been crumpled and reduced so small that we couldn't even try to smash it for access to the patient.

The only way I could access the patient was from the back window.

Coordination and communication is key with other allied services. In many motor vehicle collisions, the fire department may have to make the vehicle safe before anybody approaches. This may entail cutting the power from the vehicle, putting out fires or placing cribbing to stabilize an overturned or unbalanced vehicle.

I asked the firefighters if it was safe to climb into the vehicle, and they gave me a nod. I jumped into the bed of the truck and smashed the back window. I could only see the upper half of the driver's back, shoulders and head. I assumed he was male. His head was bent at a ninety-degree angle with his ear touching his shoulder.

This can't be good.

Nor is the fact that I can't access his airway because the speedometer was right up against his face. I cut his clothes so I could attach the cardiac monitor.

Flatline, as I expected.

The fire department told me it would be twenty minutes minimum to extricate him. With no way of doing CPR and no way of accessing the patient until extrication, I called a doctor for pronouncement. I got it pretty quickly.

I found out later that he had been at a nearby club. After leaving, he got on the exit ramp to the highway and travelled the wrong way. Then he tried to exit on an entrance ramp, which was where he met the transport truck head-on. Strangely, this was happening as my partner was telling me the story. I told her she wasn't allowed to tell me any other stories that night.

COME RIDE WITH ME

Season: Winter
Time: 0530hrs
Weather: Snow covered ground, -10°C
Area Demographic: 100km/h highway
Dispatch Info: Car into a tree

I was working the night shift at the Ancaster Fire Station, which was nostalgic for me as I'd completed my high school co-op there. A new student was riding out with me for the first time. The night was slower than usual, and by midnight, we hadn't even turned a wheel. The student was only nineteen and raring to go. I could see he was getting bored, and I was running out of stories to tell by this time, but I kept saying that you never know what might happen. By two o'clock, I knew he didn't believe me, and he was fast asleep.

At 5:30 a.m., the tones went off and woke us all out of sleep. "Motor vehicle collision, car into a tree" was the information dispatch gave us. I don't know why, but the fire department was not dispatched until five minutes later.

As we got closer to the location of the call, my partner kept a lookout on the driver's side and I kept a lookout on the passenger side. I saw tire tracks in the snow that veered off the road. The trail must have been at least half a kilometre long. It led to the car that was into a tree—and it was on fire. The flames were coming out from the hood, and smoke was just visible at the treetop level. Strangely, it looked quite pleasant in the morning against the backdrop of pine trees and snow. About one hundred metres from the highway, two male bystanders were trying to open the car door.

Paramedics are supposed to wait and let the fire department make the scene safe before initiating patient extrication, but they were five minutes behind and there wasn't a second to spare. I grabbed the defibrillator and fire extinguisher and started running towards the car. Halfway there, I fell flat on my butt and realized why we shouldn't run. I set the defibrillator down ten metres from the vehicle and looked back to see my partner and the student wheeling the stretcher out. The bystanders had opened the door, and I made a quick assessment of the patient. I determined it was an elderly male weighing about two hundred pounds. His nose was bloody, he was motionless—probably vital signs absent (VSA). I didn't see any other occupants. I looked at the floor of the car and noticed his feet were catching fire. In fact, the whole floor of the car was beginning to catch fire, and it was creating an ironic sense of warmth in the freezing cold. It also provided a bright source of light for us.

The two bystanders were having trouble undoing the seat belt, so I cut it and we dragged him out. I was out of breath by this point, and so was one of the bystanders. Panting, he suggested we get a little farther from the burning car, so we moved him another ten feet. As soon as we set him down, the vehicle erupted in a roaring fire that consumed the entire cabin.

"Good call!" I said, wide eyed.

When I finally felt safe enough to do a thorough assessment, I confirmed his vital signs were absent. Due to the long tire tracks, the amount of damage to the car and the minimal trauma to the patient, both my partner and I believed this man had a massive heart attack on the road, tried to pull off and his heart stopped.

I started CPR as the fire rescue truck arrived. I thought about using the defibrillator, but I hadn't cut his clothes off yet, I was in a ravine, and it was -10°C. I decided that it would be better to do basic airway management, CPR, immobilize and get him in the ambulance. I was getting cold as well. In my haste, I ran out without gloves, jacket or winter hat. It was early on in my career, and I had a panic factor that was difficult to control at times.

The sheer intensity of the call kept me warm enough to get him to the ambulance. On the way to the hospital, we provided full advanced cardiac life support. We shocked him multiple times and gave IV drugs to no avail. The hospital provided a passive resuscitation for a few minutes before pronouncing him. I never did see that student again; I wish him well.

Season: Summer
Time: 0200hrs
Weather: Cool, clear night, 10°C
Area Demographic: 100k/m highway
Dispatch Info: Van into a guard rail

This call initially came to the police before the collision occurred. Numerous cars had reported a cargo truck driving erratically. The patient was driving so dangerously that other drivers did not feel safe to pass it, so they all followed behind. Within a few minutes, twelve cars were following the van, including the police. They had set up a roadblock a few kilometres ahead to try and stop him, but he never made it there.

The first thing I noticed when we arrived at the scene was the steering wheel sticking out of the back of the vehicle. When we got closer, I could see it was the entire steering column. A firefighter later told me that the jaws of life were not powerful enough to cut that part from the car, so that gives you an idea of the sheer amount of force involved. The van had impaled on the guard rail like a shish kebab. The guard rail entered through the front grill and pushed the steering column out the back window. The driver's side window had unidentifiable human remains smeared on it, so it was likely if we found someone, they would be dead.

The police officer led me to the body, which was located in the ditch, ten metres ahead of the van. I had called a doc ahead of time to get an early pronouncement. There are only a few things we can call obviously dead in traumatic cases. Without going into too much detail, if their head and body are together and their insides are still inside, we begin resuscitation. This guy was very dead, but not enough for me to call it alone.

I explained to the doc that I was looking at a male in his mid-thirties who was lying on his back. His legs were torn open with multiple fractures and exposed adipose tissue. I figured this is what was smeared on the window of the van. I said that his head was pushed down into his body such that his chin was between his nipples and his ears lined up with his shoulders. His mouth was torn into four pieces that made it look like an insect's mandible. I had to lift his head off of his chest to check for a pulse. It didn't feel like a head at all—more like a mushy, rotten pumpkin. Of course, there was no pulse. The doc and I agreed there was nothing I could do. We were both glad he didn't kill anyone else.

I returned to the wreck to see if I could figure out what happened and how he ended up in front of the vehicle. The van had its roof torn open on the driver's side, and I initially didn't think it was enough for a human being to fit through. Considering how mangled the body was, this small tear in the roof was the only place the driver could have come from.

Calls like these always brought me back to high school assemblies where teachers begged us not to drink and drive. I would witness why throughout my career with examples like this.

Season: Early spring
Time: 0300hrs
Weather: Cool, crisp and clear
Area: 100km/h highway
Dispatch Info: Head-on collision

Collisions like these are as spectacular as they come. On this particular night, the police had been chasing two cars that were speeding. One was going the right way on the highway, the other was going the opposite direction. They met in the middle with catastrophic results.

Our ambulance was the second unit into the scene. As we approached, we saw one of the cars completely engulfed in flames. There were drops of fire spilling from underneath the engine onto the pavement. Everything was beginning to melt. It was against the median of the highway, so we parked on the opposite side, five lanes directly across from the flaming fireball of a car.

We were mobile from the hospital when we got the call, so we beat the fire department to the scene. As we were there first, I thought I'd unleash an extinguisher on the car.

I thought wrong.

I felt the heat on my face as soon as I got out of the ambulance—even being five lanes away! The heat was so intense I didn't feel safe coming any closer. I stood in awe as the car burned. I could see the silhouette of a human being in the driver's seat, but there was nothing I could do.

The paramedics who were on-scene first were attending to the patient from the other car. It was travelling the right way with only a single occupant. The paramedics communicated to me that they would transport the patient to the trauma centre immediately. I had to stick by in case there were any more patients. It seemed like the fire department took forever. It was the first time in my career I had to wait on-scene for an allied responder. Now I knew what it felt like to wait, and why when we showed up on-scene in five minutes, people still felt like we took forever. The fire department arrived at the scene and started to knock the flames down as they edged closer to the wreck.

As they started to get control of the flames, the damage revealed itself. There was nothing left of the car but the frame and a single occupant. The driver was behind what was left of the steering wheel, which almost touched the charred body's head. The driver's seat had been thrust back to a forty-five-degree angle, which meant that the impact of the collision had pushed the steering column right against the driver and driven the seat back. Airbag or not, the steering column would have likely struck the patient so hard in the chest that it caused a complete aortic rupture, killing them instantly. Thank god they wouldn't have endured the agony of burning to death.

As a paramedic, we have to declare the patient obviously dead. When it was all said and done, the body was so charred that only a forensic anthropologist would have been able to determine its sex. The other patient only broke both wrists, likely from the impact of the airbag. He was clocked at 150 km/hour. Due to confidentiality reasons I won't mention the make and model of his car, but I will say that the collision report was impressive.

Motor vehicle collisions (MVC) are one of the most common calls we attend. It's a chance to see the synergistic effects of all first responders in one arena—only that arena is not in an enclosed environment or anywhere predictable. That's why I refer to it as organized chaos. The next time you drive by an MVC and see a bunch of first responders looking like they are running around like chickens with their heads cut off, remember that organized chaos is taking place right before your eyes.

Chapter song selection: "Drive" by The Cars

Chapter 3

Paramedic Dilemmas

One of the things I enjoy about being a paramedic is the ability to make decisions on my own. I don't have a boss looking over my shoulder when I have to make a critical decision, and I don't have to check with a committee before going forward with a plan. We have medical directives to follow, but every patient does not fit them perfectly, so decisions have to be made outside the box. Also, the environment is dynamic and adds challenges not faced in a static emergency room. Hospitals also have a team of doctors and various medical personnel to help make decisions.

In the field, it is just me. I can bounce decisions off my partner, which I often do. In a last-ditch effort, I will phone an on-call doctor for a consultation, but for the majority of calls, I have to bear the burden of my decisions and actions. It is a double-edged sword. There have been more than a few times when I have had to make a decision that would dramatically affect the outcome. In these moments, seconds count, and making a phone call to a doctor would take too much precious time. When the pressure in the moment is palpable, you still have to take time to review the consequences of your decision. This is essential in order to have the best possible outcome to a paramedic dilemma.

Season: Summer
Time: 0000hrs
Weather: Clear, warm night, 25°C
Area Demographic: Wealthy nursing home
Dispatch Info: 94yo female, unwell, short of breath

We were dispatched to this with no lights and sirens because it was a non-emergency call. My partner and I had time to talk about our game plan on the way. Something didn't smell right. Nursing homes generally wait until the morning shift change for low priority calls that are not an emergency. Ninety-four-year-old patients have multiple illnesses that make them sicker than your average patient. If the patient is short of breath, that usually triggers a lights and sirens response. So why weren't we dispatched accordingly? I would soon find out why …

Quietly, we rolled up on the scene, and the night nurse met us at the door. In the elevator, she told us the patient had been short of breath for three days and it was getting worse. I could tell from the nurse's body language that something wasn't right. She didn't make eye contact, and her statements were short. Her bottom jaw was protruding, which to me was a sign of heighted frustration. I turned my attention to the patient's medical records. She had a "do not resuscitate" order that was valid and dated, a medical history of common illness associated with the elderly inculding congestive heart failure. The nurse pointed out a recent set of vital signs on the back of the medical records: blood pressure 189/70, heart rate 140, sp02 (oxygen saturation level) 88, respiration 40, and temp 37.0.

Okay, this spells congestive heart failure, I thought. *On paper this looks really sick—emergency sick. Why weren't we dispatched accordingly?*

What the night nurse left out was the family feud that had been raging all night.

When I entered the room, a man in his sixties greeted me, sounding very concerned.

"My mother is sick and needs to go to the hospital," he said.

He was a big man, about 6'2" and weighing 260 pounds, sharply dressed in a dark navy-blue suit. An intimidating figure. He towered over my 5'5" frame. I turned to look at the patient for a glancing assessment. She was sitting on the bed and I could see she was struggling to breathe. Her breathing rate was over 40 per minute, normal is about 20. She was using her neck muscles to breathe, and I could hear that her lungs were full of fluid. It was clear after talking with her in the first few sentences that "hospital" was not in her vocabulary. I asked her if I could take her vital signs and put a cardiac monitor on her. She nodded. Her vital signs pretty much matched the ones on the nurse's report. The son was getting impatient. He approached me abruptly, invading my personal space. He raised his voice and insisted we go to the hospital now. As sick as she was, the patient interrupted us, shook her head and repeated that she did not want to go. The son interjected and told me she was too ill to make her own decisions. I addressed her directly and looked her in the eyes. I told her if we did not go to the hospital, she would die.

"That would please me," she wheezed.

She was ready to die and was at peace with her decision.

Here's the dilemma: Whom do I fight for here?

This woman of ninety-four years clearly told me she wanted to die, and she had signed a "do not resuscitate" form confirming that. The son, a large intimidating man, sounded like he was three inches from a lawsuit and wanted me to take her against her will. My partner put oxygen on the patient while I took the son outside. I asked him if he had power of attorney, and he evaded the question by telling me what he would do to me if I didn't take his mother to the hospital. I dug my feet in and asked him until he finally said that his sister had power of attorney.

As this woman was drowning in her own lungs, she still had enough fight to say, "I'm not going. I'm dying here." I got the sister on the phone and she firmly asked to talk with her brother. With a defeated face he handed the phone to me.

"I know my mother's wishes; you leave her there please!" she said.

Thank god! I cheer to myself.

If you live to be ninety-four and want to die, who am I to stop it? This woman had dignity and no pity for herself. She was facing death and suffering with courage unbeknownst to me. I couldn't help but admire her.

As we exited, the son said, "I'm sorry. I'm used to fixing things. I can't fix this …" I couldn't be angry at a son who was watching his mother die.

Season: Summer
Time: 1256hrs
Weather: Hot, hazy and humid 30°C
Area Demographic: Industrial workplace
Dispatch Info: Patient electrocuted,
　　vital signs absent

Industrial calls are not run-of-the-mill. Depending on where you work, you could go your entire career and never attend to an industrial accident. Hamilton is a big industrial town. There are many manufacturing plants for various products. It used to be a huge steel manufacturing giant. But like all manufacturing, things slowly moved overseas. My dad worked for the steel company for thirty-eight years, and I remember him talking about how his company put safety first. This was, of course, because they had to pay out large sums of money if something went wrong.

The call came in just after lunchtime.

A single paramedic unit arrived on-scene first, and we received limited radio updates as we were en route. I recognized the voice, and there was a hint of distress. We arrived at a steel processing plant that processed flat-rolled steel. As I walked in, I was in shock as to what I saw. Thirty feet in the air, I saw Jane, a fellow paramedic, performing CPR on a man. She was in a tiny pulpit that was dropped below the crane to access a few electrical panels. The platform was about six feet long, four feet wide and six feet high. It was open on all sides and had guard rails to prevent people from falling out.

A man in a white hat greeted me and showed me the way to the suspended pulpit. I asked him if everything was locked out (all machines off and safe), and he said yes. I spent a summer working at Stelco Steel and had learned about the locking out procedure for equipment at factories. You can imagine the horror stories that come from unsafe machinery.

As I climbed a ladder and crossed the crane that spanned one hundred feet, the man told me a witness saw the patient slump over slowly and become unresponsive. I reached a tiny hatch and left my equipment on the crane. I lowered myself into the small opening, then climbed down the ladder.

By this time, my partner was behind me. I decided that there should only be two of us in the pulpit because it was too small for any more. It would be so tight that one wrong movement could knock someone to their death.

Jane was sweating profusely, and I took over CPR while trying to figure out what I was going to do. The rope rescue unit from the fire department was assembling below, and they were deciding how they were going to get this patient out. With the extremely limited space, I decided I would not try intubation because his head was right near the edge. CPR, basic airway management, defibrillation and drugs were going to have to be the focus of my treatment. I also decided we were not going to move him until we got an IV and at least one round of drugs. Since the man was working on electrical panels, Jane needed to look for exit or entry wounds for possible electrocution. We couldn't see anything obvious at the time.

"Toss down the equipment!" I yelled up to my fellow medics.

The monitor came down and I quickly applied it. Flatline. I was kneeling at the patient's right side, up into his armpit, his left arm dangling over the edge. It would have been too dangerous to start an IV in that arm, so for the first time in my career, I started an IV with my left hand.

I considered what the witness saw. The slumping over wouldn't indicate electrocution, we couldn't find evidence of electrocution and there was no smell of burnt flesh. We decided this was a medical arrest and not electrocution.

Below, an audience of approximately fifty people—staff from the plant, police, fire department—had gathered, all eyes fixed on this little pulpit. Their tension was palpable.

"We're ready to extricate," rope rescue shouted.

"How long will it take to get him to the floor?" I bounced back.

"At least twelve minutes," rope rescue replied.

The dilemma was do I stop CPR and begin extrication? This would surely seal his death as his heart hadn't started beating yet. Doing CPR is only 30 percent effective as your own heart beating, so stopping it for twelve minutes would be certain death. Should I try to get his heart started first, and if it doesn't start, pronounce him right on this pulpit? The whole audience would see me stop resuscitation on their co-worker. I didn't like this choice, but he had no chance if we went with rope extrication. If I didn't get a pulse back, there was no way this man would live.

The resuscitation went well, we attained good air entry with the bag valve mask and got his heart to show electrical activity on the monitor, but no pulse. Reluctantly, I called for a pronouncement. The doc wanted me to remove his clothing from head to toe to find a possible electrocution wound, but I declined. Leaning over to do so may have put me over the edge of the pulpit and could result in a thirty-foot drop. I got the pronouncement and we stop working on the man.

I looked down to see disappointment on the faces of the fifty-plus onlookers. I could feel it.

I had been on a single knee for about twenty minutes, and I was so stiff I couldn't get up for a couple of minutes. I was in my late thirties, so the physical tasks were becoming increasingly less comfortable. My supervisor had been watching and, thinking I was upset, put his hand on my shoulder and told me that I did a great job. When I informed him I was stiff and just couldn't get up right away, he let out a small chuckle. We were still in the public eye and had to remain professional.

I stood there for a moment and mentally went over the call. I asked my supervisor and Jane if they thought there was anything else we could have done, and we were satisfied that we did the best we could for this man. Knowing that, helps us sleep better.

Season: Fall
Time: 0800hrs
Weather: Cool and breezy, 12°C
Area Demographic: Group home for troubled teens
Dispatch Info: 17yo female cutting herself

A group home worker met me at the door and guided me upstairs to the room where the patient was and assured me that the razor had been confiscated. There was a medic already on-scene, and the patient was hiding in the closet. The medic was talking to her, calming her down. Eventually, he convinced her to come out of the closet. She had a deep laceration to her inner wrist, but the bleeding had stopped. I bandaged it and took her vital signs. They were stable, so we chit chatted with the patient, who was calm and cooperative. When the police showed up, we cleared them as the patient was cooperative. We listened to her story about what was bothering her today and let her know that we would bring her to the hospital. She didn't want to go—at all.

I know that psych hospitals sometimes don't help. In fact, I don't understand how anyone can heal in rooms that resemble a prison cell. But we have a duty of care under the mental health act for patients that are a danger to themselves. By law, we have to transport them to the hospital, so there isn't a choice whether the patient comes or not. It was just a matter of letting her down easy.

Some medics choose to be aggressive and stern with patients, but Jack and I are different. We started off being nice to let the patient know that we cared and that she needed help. After once again refusing, we informed her that she didn't have a choice. We also told her that if she refused to come voluntarily, we would have to call the police back. With the police on the way, she became more agitated. The agitation reached its peak and out came a second razor blade. We didn't know she had two. With the police on-scene first and the staff saying they removed the razor blade, we thought the scene was safe.

The dilemma was do I call on the radio for a 10-2000, which means for the police to come immediately because our lives were in danger? This would mean police speeding to the scene with lights and sirens, further agitating the patient. Leaving was an option. We could try to disarm the patient, but things could go wrong, and it's harder to explain on paper why you made that choice. Jack and I are good conversationalists, so we decided to try and talk her down.

She held the blade up like a card, examining it. We watched every move she made just in case she attacked. A single officer arrived and was wide-eyed when he saw the blade. This officer did not have a taser, so he put his hand on his gun. With his other hand up in a pleading position, he calmly said, "I don't want to hurt anybody today, so please give up the razor."

"Listen, we don't need another statistic," I begged. "We really want you to come and get help."

She slowly gave it up and everyone breathed a sigh of relief.

I still wonder to this day what I would have done if she started carving herself up or attacked us. Later, that police officer thanked us; he didn't want to shoot someone that day. Most police services place you on administrative leave if you are involved in a shooting.

"Administrative leave isn't as appealing as it sounds," I said to the officer.

He gave me a slow nod.

Season: Early spring
Time: 2100hrs
Weather: Cool and crisp, no precipitation
Area Demographic: Urban core
Dispatch Info: 3yo choking. No further information

I've done a bunch of these calls. Typically, we get there and the crying is audible from outside the house. The parents are hysterical, and there is an object like candy on the floor, and the patient is fine. This particular time, we rolled up to a house on a small dead-end street. Cars were parked on both sides of the road, making it impossible to make a turn on the street with the ambulance. My partner and I decided to park on the corner and walk to the house, which was only three houses in. The fire department went in first. We enter the house, and it is alarmingly quiet.

"Ambulance!" my partner yelled.

We don't hear a thing.

"Where are you guys?" I shouted.

"Upstairs!"

On the second floor, I peer over the railing into one of the bedrooms. What I see is something I was not prepared for. The fire department was starting CPR on a little three-year-old girl.

I was not prepared for this for a few reasons. First, we did not get an update from dispatch that the patient was VSA, and the call information said nothing about the patient being unconscious. Second, the fire department did not call out that the patient was VSA, which they usually do. Anyhow, it was time to kick it into sixth gear—one I don't use very often.

"We can't get the airway in, and there is a lot of stuff in her mouth," the fire captain said. "We can't get a pulse either."

The mother was sitting on the bed watching as we tried to save her little girl's life, and I got a bit of a story as I unloaded my equipment. She was heard choking on the second floor, her siblings were watching her and called for mom. The mother tried to remove the obstruction herself but was unable to do so.

I started basic airway management and used a finger sweep to remove what looked like white styrofoam. Thinking I had removed the obstruction, we tried to ventilate but did not get any signs that air was moving into her lungs. Then, because of CPR, a copious amount of vomit came up, so we suctioned what we could. I got my laryngoscope out and tried to view the obstruction that I knew was more profound than we could see. I positioned the handle of my scope to see the vocal cords, but I couldn't. All I saw was white, murky styrofoam. (I couldn't identify the substance.)

The dilemma was that I had been on the scene for some time and knew I should transport as soon as possible. But to get her to the ambulance, we had to take her downstairs and outside. This would certainly limit her chances of survival if we did not have her airway cleared and secured. So would spending too much time on-scene getting an airway in place.

I call this getting task focused. It's a mistake paramedics make when they cannot complete an important task, spend too much time on it and fail to move on. It can drastically change the outcome of a patient.

I thought of my kids and what would I do if it were them. I decided I wouldn't leave until I gave it my best shot at getting an airway.

This was one of the most stressful situations I had been in during my almost twenty years on the job. I felt the intense pressure with the mother still watching. I pulled out the murky white substance from deep in her mouth, the oropharynx and even between the vocal cords. There were also pieces beyond the vocal cords that I was not able to get. I intubated the little girl and finally got some air in after eight minutes or so of resuscitation. The reading from the carbon dioxide detector confirmed that the tube was in the right place, in trachea not the esophagus. Now we could finally get going to the hospital. Thank god it was only two minutes away.

The nearest hospital wasn't a pediatric facility, but the medical profession goes the extra mile for children; it's a privilege to witness. All hands were on deck when we got there—there must have been fifteen medical personnel in that room helping out.

After I was done handing over and giving a report, I needed a break. I got a coffee from the café that was always open and then cleaned the back of the ambulance, which looked like a tornado had hit it. After about half an hour, I came back. They were still working on the little girl. Mom was brought in to watch. I was told that it was best that the parents are present during the resuscitation so they can see that everything was being done.

Finally, after an hour, the doctor walked up to tell the mother the news she already knew. Knowing it is coming doesn't soften the blow. I watched as she looked at the floor as the doctor approached her. He explained that they had tried everything, but it hadn't worked. With his hand on her shoulder he told her that her child was dead. She sobbed as her friend consoled her. That was final for me. As hard as it was to watch, it was closure. I needed to know that no matter what I did, I couldn't make it better. The hospital staff couldn't make it better. No one could make it better. And that's just the way it goes sometimes.

My supervisor asked if I needed to go home, and I said I'd complete my paperwork and then decide. It was the night shift, and it did not make sense to me to go home. Everybody would be asleep, and all I'd do is lie awake dwelling on things, trying to be quiet. So, I finished my paperwork and did a few more calls before I went home. The last call put me into overtime, but it was an elderly man who really needed help. His blood pressure had dropped so low he passed out and couldn't stand up. I remember being glad I stayed because I got to help one more person that night. Someone who had a positive outcome.

Tired and emotionally exhausted, I headed home. I peered into my three-year-old daughter's room and watched her sleep peacefully, thankful for everything I had.

There would be no challenge or responsibility without dilemmas in our profession. It's something that comes easier with experience. On her last day, one of my best advanced care paramedic students asked me for advice.

"Prepare for the worst, hope for the best, keep it simple if you can, and always look before you leap," I said.

It's the template I will continue to use in any paramedic dilemma.

Chapter song selection:
"Choices" by George Jones.

Chapter 4

The Mentally Ill

Responding to patients with a mental illness makes up a significant portion of our call volume. During the first few years of my career, I loathed going to these calls because I felt they were not worthy of a paramedic attending. My mind changed as the years went by. With more life experience, I had the patience and empathy to deal with people who were in serious trouble. Mental illness is extremely underfunded and is often misunderstood. As a society we have attached a negative stigma to it. I learned to be more empathetic on these calls, and I experienced better patient outcomes.

We never know what to expect: suicide, depression, dementia, hallucinations, schizophrenia, delusions, paranoia, personality disorders, anxiety, excited delirium and hypochondria are just a few of the challenges people face. Back when I went to school, there wasn't any comprehensive training on how to treat these patients and their underlying mental illnesses, so I learned on the job. I found that being kind and listening actively has produced a positive outcome in most cases.

Season: Spring
Time: 1300hrs
Weather: Cool, 10°C
Area Demographic: Apartment building on a wealthy side of town
Dispatch Info: Elderly male, erratic behaviour

We were greeted by an intensely frustrated woman at the door of the apartment who insisted her husband was acting bizarrely. She told us that he had urinated in the dresser drawer, poured milk into a vase and talked to a chair.

Dementia for sure, I thought to myself.

Her husband was sitting on the bed not speaking. He looked spaced-out, confused and lost. After a thorough assessment we found him to be displaying dementia-like behaviour, and his wife confirmed that he had recently been diagnosed. She also rambled angrily about how she could not leave the apartment to go grocery shopping for fear of him doing something erratic. I asked her if his behaviour was getting worse or if anything had changed recently. She denied any change in behaviour but insists that he needed to go to the hospital. I asked if she had someone that could help her or watch him when she went out. She looked down at the floor and shook her head. She conveyed that she had been taking care of him in this state for five years. She started to cry, and with a commanding voice insisted that she still loved him but he was not the same person anymore.

I softened my voice and commended her for taking care of him for so long. I agreed that he was not the same person he once was, and that man she loved had changed. I explained that it was not that she didn't love him anymore but that she was experiencing caregiver burnout. She denied it and expressed that she had no problem taking care of him.

"Then why are we here?" I gently asked.

She started to cry again and I put my hand on her shoulder and let her know it was okay to need a break. My partner and I gave her the contact information for various community resources which could provide her with some in-home care.

About a month later, my supervisor contacted me to say that the woman from that call stopped him at the hospital and told him that I saved her life. She had arranged for home care and was doing so much better. The frustration and resentment were gone because she was getting some time for herself. It was nice to help someone in a different way.

This call would come back into my subconscious many times over the years. When my uncle passed away, I was left with the task of taking care of my aunt who had Parkinson's dementia. With a family of my own to take care of, it was hard to take care of her as well. Eventually, I got her into a great nursing home where my daughter and I regularly visited. I always kept this woman in mind when I got frustrated with how much time my aunt took up, and it made me lead by example.

Season: Winter
Time: 1420hrs
Weather: Cold, -5°C
Area Demographic: Urban core
Dispatch Info: Elderly male trying to jump out of a window; possible excited delirium

My level of awareness goes up when I hear these calls. They are usually pretty intense and can get quite physical. As we approached, we saw that police were on-scene and already up in the attic apartment. It was a three-storey walk-up with a rickety, narrow metal staircase. After opening the door to the attic apartment, I was greeted with an unusual scene. There was a naked elderly man, 5'3", one hundred pounds, fighting with two police officers, one who is 6'6". The little man was giving them a run for their money, screaming at the top of his lungs like a banshee and flailing about with the energy of an eighteen-year-old.

"I don't want to hurt him!" the tall officer keeps repeating as they struggle to get handcuffs on this man.

This gained my utmost respect. At his size, in an enclosed environment with no outside witnesses, he could have chosen to use brute force and harm this man. Instead, he tried to help the patient.

As the naked man squirmed like a little worm, I jumped into action. While the two officers were trying to put the cuffs on, I grabbed his legs, similar to a double-leg takedown, which made it easier for the officers. The officers sat him down on a chair and, even with the handcuffs on, he was still screaming and flailing about like his life was in danger.

My field diagnosis pointed to a case of excited delirium. This frequently involves drug use but can arise from mental illness alone. Either way, fatalities can occur. The best way I can explain excited delirium is that your body is operating well above the red line on your personal tachometer. If the engine of a car revs above the red line for too long, it will fail. Likewise, a body cannot operate at these levels for too long before sudden cardiac arrest occurs. So intervention is required. The treatment is sedation with Midazolam or ketamine, medications that can knock them out cold … most of the time.

I jabbed the patent in the leg with the medication. Drugs affect people differently, and it took a long time for this man. We got a pair of shorts on him and the police escorted him to the staircase. He got a boost of energy and wrapped his legs around one of the support posts, but after a few minutes, the drug finally took effect. His eyes got heavy and his legs relaxed. Finally, he walked down the rickety staircase on his own accord. At the bottom, he offered one more act of defiance and refused to get on the stretcher. The tall officer picked the man up by his shoulders like he was a boy and placed him on the stretcher. With that, I wrapped the man in a blanket and he fell fast asleep. He stayed asleep all the way to the hospital.

With all the flack about police brutality, it was nice to know there were police officers that were non-judgemental and treated that man like a patient and not a criminal. Acts like these go unappreciated, and undocumented.

Season: Fall
Time: 1850hrs
Weather: Cool, 12°C
Area Demographic: Suburban community with farms and vineyards
Dispatch Info: Mass burial site

"Dispatch can you repeat that?" I said into the radio.

"You're going to a mass burial site. The person who made the report is going to meet you on Plantation Road about halfway down southbound between Warlock and Highway 7. It's a male with a black coat and blonde hair. That's all the info we have."

Well, I've never heard of anything like this going across the radio waves before. I hope this is not true, as I think I may need a long vacation after this call. What will I do if we actually find a mass burial site?

I didn't have the answers at the time, so I concentrated on driving to the call. I was slightly confused as to what a couple of medics and an ambulance were supposed to do for this situation, but I was about to find out as we approached the scene.

Coming up the road that dispatch told us, I saw a man fitting the description. We shut the lights and sirens off and I rolled down the window. Choosing my words carefully, I asked the man if he called in an emergency. The man walked with conviction and purpose, looked at me seriously and commanded me to follow him. I didn't want to ask him about the burial site directly or agitate him, but after a few minutes, I finally asked where we were going.

"You'll see! Oh, you'll see!" he said with wide eyes.

We walked about half a kilometre and he led us into a small field on somebody's property. He then got very emotional and started to sigh and breathe heavily. Holding his heart, he began to whimper. With his hands making circular motions, he revealed we were in the mass burial site. Although I thought we were just in a small field, I did not want to lose this man's trust or agitate him. We took him seriously and indulged his endeavours. As we walked, he pointed to a decrepit old tractor in the field and said that was a marker for the site.

That it is just a tractor, nothing special about it, I think to myself.

We walked towards it and eventually came to a canvas tarp on the ground. Again, he got emotional and started to whimper as he pointed to the tarp and motioned for me to lift it up.

"What will I find?" I asked politely.

"A dead body," he stated with conviction.

I admit that a part of me was freaking out, worried that I would, in fact, find a dead body underneath the tarp. The tarp was made of canvas, and I could tell it had been there for a long time. This call happened well before the residential schools were in the news, so there was no way he could have been influenced by them.

To my relief, when I lifted the tarp, there was not a body underneath. Just cold hard ground. The man looked confused and assured me that the next place would have a dead body. We searched two more sites and, thankfully, found no carcasses. I was careful what I said to the man, as he clearly believed what he was telling us. I apologized that we couldn't find anything, and at no time did I act like I did not believe him.

The police arrived, and I asked him if there was anything we could help him with or if there was somebody he would like to talk to. He admitted that he was stressed and wanted to go home. The police and I suggested he go to the hospital to talk to somebody about his strange beliefs. He agreed and decided to go with the police. As he left with one officer, I asked the other officer what he would have done if we actually found a mass burial site.

"Book off," he joked.

Season: Summer
Time: 1830hrs
Weather: Warm, sunny, 20°C
Area Demographic: East end
Dispatch Info: 20yo male, bizarre behaviour on the bus

The base pager went off as soon as we entered the door for shift change, so we hopped in the ambulance and raced off. As we approached the bus, I saw two police cruisers on-scene, which made us feel a little safer. I stepped inside the bus and the officer said that the original complaint which came to police was about a passenger who would not get off the bus. When the police went to interview him, they realized he was acting strange and not answering questions appropriately. So, we were dispatched to see if there was a medical explanation for this.

I sized the patient up as I approached him. It's a safety thing. You never know when these patients are going to snap. He was 5'4", 180 pounds, and looked a little scruffy. I sensed, as Jason Bourne might say, "He can handle himself." Since we had two police officers on-scene, it felt safe to approach.

As I started talking to the patient, I noticed he wouldn't make eye contact. He was staring over my right shoulder without blinking. When answering questions, most of his responses were scattered and not on the topic that was asked.

"What medications are you on?" I asked.

"They are coming," he answered.

He seemed to have a preoccupation with "they," and no matter how I asked about "them," he would never tell me who "they" were. During this bizarre conversation, his tone was passive and his voice was soft. He denied any drug use that day and his breath didn't smell like alcohol, so I was at a loss for what was causing this bizarre behaviour other than a psychotic episode. For this reason and the patient's safety, the police decided he would be apprehended and transported to the hospital for an assessment.

But first, we had to get him off the bus.

I convinced him that we would have a better conversation about "them" if we were outside the bus. I also threw out that the weather was so nice we had to enjoy it. Humour is a tool I constantly use to lighten difficult situations. He came off the bus and his body language changed as soon as he noticed the stretcher. His chest puffed out, he stood more erect and the tone of his voice changed to aggressive and angry.

I'd fought competitively in karate tournaments for fifteen years, and there was always "that guy" who was a little crazy and just out to hurt people. I got the same feeling about this guy. I pulled the officers aside and told them we would likely have a problem when we went to put him on the stretcher, and we devised a plan to take him safely without hurting him.

Each of the two officers took a hand and started to guide the patient to the stretcher. He began to resist violently, first by kicking us. I grabbed a leg, my partner grabbed the other leg and we got him on the stretcher. He was so strong it took us all to hold him down. I got a high Brazilian jiu-jitsu mount on him—I was sitting on his chest with my knees high up in his armpits. This was not to hurt him but to control him and prevent him from hurting himself and others.

I had a dose of Midazolam ready and injected him in the shoulder. It took a few minutes to kick in but eventually rendered him unconscious and snoring. We all breathed a sigh of relief and transported him to the hospital without incident. Later that night, we found out that his drug toxicology was negative for most of the common street drugs. Psych would come and evaluate him the next day. I didn't follow up on his final psychiatric diagnosis, as it is hard to find out once they leave the emergency department. I was just glad we were able to sedate him without hurting him. It would have looked terrible to the people standing on the street beside the bus.

During my career I've had to become increasingly aware of people filming us. When I started, digital recording devices were low resolution and expensive. Now you can whip out your phone and make a movie anywhere. It's something I'm glad I kept in mind during this call.

Mental illness continues to rise in our communities. What was once a shameful diagnosis is becoming more accepted, but we aren't where we need to be with it. It frustrates me to no end to see the same patients day in and out not getting the help they need. But as the saying goes, it's out of my control and above my pay grade. So I'll do what I can by educating myself and keeping a positive attitude when faced with these situations.

Chapter song selection:
"People Are Strange" by The Doors

Chapter 5

Fire

If you can't stand the heat, stay out of the kitchen and don't become a firefighter. I was lucky enough to have a firefighting co-op in high school. Lights and sirens, holding that nozzle and saving the day are what I thought firefighting was all about. *Backdraft* was one of my favourite movies back then, and it was my dream to become a firefighter.

During my co-op they put me through a recruitment simulation, and I found out I couldn't fulfill my dream because I was colour blind. I also failed the physical miserably and needed to put on some serious muscle if I was going to even think about applying. I was pretty disappointed about the whole ordeal.

When you're eighteen and have your dreams crushed, it seems like the world has ended. As time passed, I became more comfortable with my decision to become a paramedic. Eventually, I would never look back as I knew I had found my calling.

The truth about fires is that they are more dangerous and frightening than I imagined. Scorching heat and smoke causing complete darkness are enough to make the best of us cower. I often responded to fires that made me thankful I never became a firefighter.

Season: Summer
Time: 1300hrs
Weather: Hot, hazy and humid, 30°C
Area Demographic: Urban core
Dispatch Info: Explosion, fire, facial burns

I was a single man unit that day and the second unit dispatched to this call. There were many updates coming across the radio as I made my way to the scene. Dispatch relayed that there was an accident involving propane tanks and flash fire.

"Is there an active fire?" I inquired.

"No active fire," dispatch replied.

Not having to worry about that put me at ease. Upon arrival, the fire department directed me to the patient. As we made our way there, one of the firefighters pointed out a pile of old propane tanks and a pile of tanks that were cut and stacked neatly in quarters. He told me that the patient was cutting them with some type of power saw and it created a flash fire. He was lucky it didn't explode.

I finally made my way to the patient and he was already loaded into the ambulance. As I was assessing him, he explained that he was cutting propane tanks for scrap metal because it was easier to transport them on his bicycle trailer. He forgot to drain one of them completely and it ignited as soon as he made it through the metal. He also admitted to using cocaine that day. I assured him there was no judgement in the back of the ambulance and I would try to take care of some of his pain soon.

His burns were concentrated to the upper torso above his chest and face and seemed to be only second degree. We started treating him by cooling the wounds with saline and then dressing them. As I looked at his face, I noticed that the skin around his eyes was not burned and his eyebrows were intact. People who get facial flash burns usually have their eyebrows singed off.

"Hey man, were you wearing safety glasses?" I asked.
"Yeah!" he replied.

It struck me as funny that in all the ridiculousness that happened in this incident, he still had the intelligence to wear safety glasses. It saved his sight. But I'm not sure his wisdom metre is anywhere near half full. Nonetheless, I gave him some morphine on the way in to ease his pain.

Season: Fall
Time: 1830hrs
Weather: Clear, cool, 15°C
Area Demographic: Maximum security prison
Dispatch Info: Fire inside the prison

It was a half hour before the end of shift and James and I really wanted to head home after a relentlessly busy day. We hadn't had a break in eleven hours and were exhausted.

One superstitious thing paramedics do is never plan anything or promise to be somewhere after work.

Murphy's Law never fails. I hate that guy …

The radio cracked to life and dispatch reported that a prison is on fire and there are multiple patients. James and I looked at the time—so much for going home on schedule. Our unit would be the first one in which meant we would have to triage the patients. Multi-casualty incidents are usually chaotic, and I have never been to one that ran smoothly. With only minutes to get there, my mind raced considering the burns and smoke inhalation injuries we would find, and I mentally pictured where the burn kit was in the back of the ambulance.

The guards opened the giant iron gate that separated us from convicted criminals. The interior of the prison was desolate, unwelcoming concrete—an interior decorator's worst nightmare. Upon entering the scene, the fire department waved us in and assured us that the scene was safe. We went through the foyer of the prison and found over thirty people packed in a room about the size of a two-car garage. The atmosphere was frantic. Sound was bouncing off the concrete walls creating a cacophony of voices. We could smell the fumes of the fire—a smell I was very familiar with by this point in my career. A hazy fog covered the entire area.

James and I got to work.

I guess a fire presents a great escape opportunity because five prisoners were being held down by guards. I approached one of the prisoners who was coughing, assuming that he needed medical attention. Out of professional respect, I asked the guard if he needed medical attention, and the guard said no. I made eye contact with the prisoner and gave him a thumbs up while asking him if he was okay. He nodded. I looked over three prisoners intently and saw they were not visibly burned and were breathing well. They all declined medical attention, which surprised me as I had transported many patients from the prison and usually they are eager to go. I also asked the staff guards if they needed medical attention; they declined.

I reconvened with James to see how sick the patients that he triaged were. He pointed out the sickest patient, a man who was unconscious and his face covered in soot. The stench of smoke was all over him, and we noted that he had soot in his nose. This told us he had inhaled smoke and was at high risk for impaired oxygen exchange. We quickly administered a treatment of salbutamol and oxygen and his breathing eased. We found out later that this patient started the fire deliberately to get the guards to respond to his cell so that he could cause some mayhem. Nonetheless, we have a duty of care in Ontario to treat patients. No discrimination for what they have done. None.

Season: Winter
Time: 0351hrs
Weather: Cold, -5°C
Area Demographic: Urban core
Dispatch Info: Person on fire

James and I had just arrived at the hospital with a non-emergent patient when we heard a call on our radio.

"2075, you're going for … um … a man reported on fire outside of 2376 Howitzer Street. Cross street of Wade Ave."

My partner and I shot each other a look. We both knew that that address was right around the corner and that the patient would be coming to this hospital since it was the regional trauma and burn centre. I gave the triage nurse a heads-up that she was probably getting a severely burned patient.

"We need a backup unit, this patient is burned real bad and combative!" the on-scene paramedic radioed, distress in his voice.

The triage nurse heard the radio transmission and made eye contact with me.

"Is your patient stable?" she asked.

"Yes, epigastric pain with a clear ECG," I replied.

"Put your patient in the waiting room and get going," the nurse said.

Usually, the triage nurse takes a report before assigning a place for the patient to go, but this nurse knew that I liked jumping on critical calls and that we were the closest unit. James and I rushed to the scene.

It took us less than two minutes to get there. As we approached, we saw the house completely engulfed in flames. The fire was rolling out of control and the flames were thirty feet in the air. Brilliant and strangely beautiful oranges and yellows emanated from the centre of the fire.

My friend and colleague on the scene tended to the patient on the sidewalk right in front of the fire. As I got out of the truck, I could see that the patient was combative, and the crew was having a hard time getting him on the stretcher.

As I jumped in to help, I witnessed the organized chaos that is firefighting. There was already a hose charged and attacking the front door, which had flames billowing out of it. Other fire crews were setting up secondary lines and the perimeter, so I tried not to get in the way as I reached the patient.

When I was about six metres from the crew, they told me the patient was found on the grass, so we don't know how he got there. The first thing the crew noted was that he was split on his left torso from his flank to his umbilicus, so they thought he may have jumped from the window. They decided to collar and board him, a practice that is no longer done.

We were less than five metres from the door and the fire was so hot that it was searing my eyeballs. I couldn't look directly at the fire for more than a second, and I had trouble keeping them open.

"Hey guys, let's get to the truck, it's too hot," I suggested.

The patient was so severely burned, I knew he would not survive the night. His eyelids were burned shut and he was writhing in pain. He couldn't make any sounds because I was sure his vocal cords were burned. His fingers and toes each had a bone protruding at the tips. His skin was like leather and was taught like a roasted pig. He had third-degree burns on most of his body. I didn't waste time with the rule of nines to estimate the body surface area that was burned—it was too much. This was one of those times where good old fashioned fast driving was the best therapy we could provide.

Considering the proximity to the trauma centre, there was no way I had time to treat his burns other than to cover him with a dry, sterile burn sheet. I got an IV line and we used our bag-valve-mask to breathe for him. In two minutes, we were at the trauma centre, and they were ready for us. Before I could even give a report to the doc, pain medication was ordered through the IV I started. Thank god, I can't imagine how much pain and suffering this man was going through. In the two minutes that we had in the back during transport, I desperately wanted to give him morphine but didn't have time.

I inquired about the massive split on his side. The trauma leader said that it was likely from the severe burns. He explained that as the burns go from degree to degree, the skin becomes less elastic. As the inside tissues burn and heat up, they expand against the now rigid skin.

"Like a sausage splitting when being cooked," he said.

I was told they would do all they could to make him comfortable but he would not last the night.

I went to get coffee. At this particular hospital, you pick up a phone to access the shop after hours. I told security that it was a medic getting a coffee.

"YEAH, THAT'S ALL YOU LAZY MEDICS DO IS GET COFFEE!" a guy behind me in the hallway yelled.

"Hey, what's wrong?" I asked.

"Where were you when my friend was burning to death?" he shouted.

I couldn't even get another word out before he hit me with a barrage of four-letter adjectives focussed on how useless I was. I stood and took it without countering because I know when I can't make a situation better. This was obviously one of the friends of my recent patient. After his verbal assault, I simply said, "I'm sorry," and went to get my coffee.

Later we learned that the patient went in to grab something of value after the fire had started. He ran out and collapsed on the sidewalk. These are things that as a medic you are not privileged to on scene. That's why we have to make the best decisions we can with what time and information we get on scene.

James and I offered to do this call because we liked to help and welcomed the challenge of a difficult call. I talked to the crew on scene and we were satisfied that we did well despite what the guy in the hallway thought.

Season: Fall
Time: 2320hrs
Weather: Cool, 12°C
Area Demographic: Urban core
Dispatch Info: House fire, possibly seven patients

It was eleven-thirty and I'd had to take a number two for the past two calls. Our service was unusually busy that night with critically ill patients. Dispatch informed us we were the last ambulance available for the region, so I'd only have a few minutes to go do my business. The hospital was the closest washroom, and I make haste. While finally getting relief, I received a text from my partner.

"House fire, multiple patients. Sounds legit … and bad."

I finished up as quickly as I could and briskly made it out to the ambulance. We sped off and dispatch gave us some disturbing news.

"4380, there are possibly seven patients, two confirmed vital signs absent, and we don't have any ambulances to send you."

My partner clicked the mic, "Copy, situation normal."

James and I discussed how messed up this is.

How can we have no backup with seven patients?

Like always, the game plan is to wing it as best we can. There's the way that you're supposed to run multi-casualty incidents, then there's the reality.

We rolled up on the scene and saw smoke billowing out the back of the house. Firefighters on-scene directed us to one of the patients that made it out. James and I set up a triage and treatment area, and James started treating that patient right away. I asked the fire captain where the VSA patients are and he says one is being brought out to us.

It seemed like a long time before the first patient arrived, and later, I read in the news how the firefighter carried the man out of the house in pitch black. He was feeling around the walls and couldn't see anything. That is what was taking so long.

I'm on the front lawn of the house, ready for the first patient.

Two firefighters carried the victim to me and we started to work on him. I had a team of firefighters to help me. I gave my phone to my supervisor to call the base hospital physician for some guidance, and he stayed on the phone while I worked on the first VSA patient.

His face was covered in soot, and as I intubated him, his airway was entirely black. Burnt human flesh has a particular smell, one you never forget. I got the order from my supervisor to cease resuscitation if there was no response after three rounds of drugs. It took me six minutes to deliver the drugs, and then we stopped. Just before I got to the end of my treatment, they brought out the second VSA patient. My supervisor got that victim pronounced right away. The first ambulance finally rolled up on the scene and took the patient that James was taking care of.

The fire captain approached me and said there was a third patient in the house that was too charred to remove—melted into the couch frame, he said. We weren't permitted to enter and have a look because it was too dangerous and they were still putting the fire out.

That meant I could take a breather. I gathered my equipment and threw it into the back of the ambulance. My hair and uniform smelled like house fire, and there was even soot in my hair. I was also sweating from the stress and physical work from the resuscitation.

My supervisor congratulated us on a job well done and then gives us the grim news that the service is still low on ambulances. James and I cleaned up as quickly as we could and spent the rest of the night doing back-to-back calls.

Exhausted and hungry, we were having a bad night. Then we responded to a girl in a family shelter who had a fever and weakness. There was a noticeable insect bite on her leg, which looked like a tick bite. It was my partner's turn to attend, so I drove with the girl's father sitting with me up front. Through casual conversation, I found out the family was from the Middle East and had only been in Canada for two weeks. The father was an engineer there, and when I asked him what made him leave, he stared me dead in the eye and replied, "When ISIS beheads somebody on your doorstep, it's time to leave."

Suddenly, we weren't having a bad night.

Fire calls still bring a level of stress in me that is above the average call. The difference is that, with growing experience, the calls get easier and less stressful. But the fragrances and images that these calls produce will be with us paramedics long after we retire.

Chapter song selection:
"The Show Goes On" by Bruce Hornsby & The Range (from the *Backdraft* soundtrack)

Chapter 6

Unpalatable Places

Paramedics never know what is beyond that barrier that separates the outside world from theirs. Until that door is open, there are only clues—demographics, odours, how the outside is kept—that help us predict what we are going to encounter. Occasionally, we have to enter an environment that is unimaginably putrid. Houses and apartments that are so inhabitable that most rational human beings would never set foot in them. As a paramedic in Ontario, we have a duty of care to treat patients, so no matter how unpalatable a dwelling may be, we have to go in.

COME RIDE WITH ME

Season: Fall
Time: 1825hrs
Weather: Cool, clear 8°C
Area Demographic: Apartment building, urban core
Dispatch Info: 55yo male, unable to ambulate

The building's superintendent met us in the lobby and informed us that he tried to evict the person. While trying to remove him, he noticed that the occupant was extremely confused, so he called us. With an arrogant smile on his face, he added that he shut off the water and electricity to the apartment. That bothered me. I was in my early twenties and thought that this landlord had too much satisfaction in his voice. With that comment, he disappeared down the hall. I looked at my partner and we both shook our heads.

How malevolent is this landlord? I thought to myself.

But as soon as we made patient contact, I forgot about the landlord and had to concentrate on the medical challenge ahead.

The apartment was dark and barely lit except for a few flashlights on the floor. It had no furniture. The only thing I could make out were endless empty twenty-four-bottle beer boxes stacked up almost to the ceiling. My partner and I saw the patient holding a flashlight and lying on the floor against a wall. We got closer and noticed he was very short of breath. He was in a puddle of his own feces, most of which had dried out. A trail of it led to the bathroom. A ratty old shirt was the only thing he was wearing. As my partner knelt beside the patient, he knocked over a bottle that turned out to be full of urine.

The foul smell hit me within seconds and I gagged before quickly regaining control of my nausea.

We put a sheet on the floor to lift the patient to our stretcher. As my partner whipped the sheet over his legs, something flipped into my mouth. Considering where the sheet had been, there were only a few possibilities. I ran to the bathroom and found that the trail of feces ended at the toilet. It was also covered in the same stuff. I chose to spit in the sink, and rinse my mouth out with hand sanitizer.

I still had a patient to take care of that was very sick, so back to the stretcher I went. My partner had him loaded up and ready to go. We provided oxygen therapy on the way to the hospital and his breathing improved.

I had a freak out at the hospital and got tested for everything. I was cleared six months later but still had to tell the embarrassing story every time I gave blood for another half year.

Season: Summer
Time: 1210hrs
Weather: Hot, humid 32°C
Area Demographic: Subsidized housing
Dispatch info: 68yo female, unresponsive

The call took us to a large townhouse complex. We had to park the ambulance on the street and walk the stretcher to get to the townhouse unit. On the way, a large man wearing a tank top and baseball cap sitting outside his house nodded to us. I humoured him and nodded back.

We arrived at the patient's house, and another man met us outside and told us that he cannot wake his mother. I could smell his body odour from a few feet away. The shirt he was wearing was white at one point, but now it was grey. He was wearing ripped jogging pants that had an underlying greyish hue with layers of brown stains. Turning around, he led us into the townhome that had its own stench. A quick glance at the condition of the place was alarming. It was a hoarding house, and there were piles of junk everywhere—open cans of food and half-eaten plates of what used to be food had varying amounts of mould on them. They covered both the kitchen table and counter. The floor was littered with garbage.

Suddenly, a little Shih Tzu popped out from one of the garbage piles, wagging its tail. I felt sorry for the little thing, but at least it appeared happy. The dog snuggled up against my boot for a quick second as we started descending the stairs to the basement.

The patient was in a chair at the bottom of the stairs. We determined that her blood sugar was low, and after an IV and sugar directly into her veins, she woke up and apologized for the mess. I hadn't had a look around the basement yet, but I took a few seconds to take things in. What stood out the most were three round, overflowing ashtrays. The mound of butts was four inches high in each of them. At the base of each of the ashtrays was a ring of more butts.

Amazed more than disgusted, I re-focused on the patient. She was wearing a diaper that was on the verge of disintegrating. It looked like it was a week old. Concerned, I asked why she is wearing it. She said that her legs had been weak for a month and she hadn't been able to walk or get up. Her son had been trying to take care of her, but his limited abilities could only do so much. Despite her not wanting to go to the hospital, I convinced her to come. Since she couldn't walk, we had to get the stair chair, an extrication device that folds up like a lawn chair and is specially made to navigate stairs, to get her out.

I needed a break from the filth and stench, so I volunteered to go get it. On my way back from the ambulance, the man with the tank top who nodded to me earlier stopped me.

"Okay man, how bad is it in there? Cause they asked me to help them move something for them, and I got three feet from the door and almost puked from the stench," the man says.

"Sir, you don't even want to know," I replied.

I got the equipment from the ambulance and a few breaths of fresh air.

Back in the basement, we loaded her onto the stair chair. There was a pile of black, dried-out feces on the spot where she was sitting. Relief washed over me that I was removing this person from this environment. I made a mental note to get social work involved at the hospital so this poor woman could get some care.

We wrapped her in a sheet like a mummy and put her on the stair chair. She was a little apprehensive about it, and she reached out to grab the handrails. I advised her to keep her hands in and reassured her that we only drop people on days other than this one. I had the bottom of the chair, and my partner took the top and we began to lift her up the stairs. About one-quarter of the way up, the sheet was displaced from her wriggling about, so I now had a view of her crotch. The diaper had broken open, and all I saw was black, rotting feces. As much as I wanted to turn away, I couldn't because I had to look up in case something fell my way. So I stared at it all the way up the stairs.

I made sure to relay the unsuitable living conditions to social work at the hospital, which was the best thing I could do for that patient. Sometimes it's not the medicine that is the greatest healer, it's the empathy for a patient.

Season: Fall
Time: 1400hrs
Weather: Warm, sunny 14°C
Area Demographic: House converted to an apartment
Dispatch Info: Man barricaded

Why am I going to this call? I thought as I hustled towards the scene.

Dispatch didn't give us any medical complaints in the info but told us police were already on the scene. Upon arrival, the cops met us outside and gave us an update on the situation.

The landlord had called the police because the man in his apartment hadn't paid rent for three months and wouldn't leave. When the cops got there, they couldn't open the door more than four inches. Upon conversing with the patron, the police determined that he was extremely confused. Also, from the direction of his voice, they thought he was against the door. His confusion was why we were called.

"Sir? Are you hurt?" I yelled through the door.

"My chair is over there," he answered.

"Can you open the door for us?" I asked.

"My dog," he answered.

These inappropriate answers to my questions confirmed how confused he was. I opened the door a couple of inches and peered in. It looked like a landfill! There was hoarding stacked six feet high that covered the entire apartment. Insects were buzzing all around and it smelled worse than a sewer.

I went back to the ambulance and put on a full isolation suit. Returning to the barricaded door, I squeezed through the four inches that were available, trying to avoid tripping on the garbage. The patient was lying on his right side, curled up in a ball. His feet were right against the door, which was why we couldn't open it. He occupied the only floor space in the entire apartment. He was naked and had long, dishevelled brown hair. He was at least 250 pounds. His lower legs were black, possibly necrotic, his blood pressure was low and he was confused. I couldn't treat or assess him any further due to the confined space. With garbage piled so high, it was tough to move and treat this patient. I observed five species of insects around him—the common housefly, earwigs, ants, a beetle and cockroaches. Extrication was imperative. Moreover, I did not want to spend more time there than I had to.

Finally, the fire department had arrived to help with the door issue.

"Do you want us to break it down?" they asked.

"No, I'm right behind it and can't move. Just gimmie a flathead screwdriver and hammer," I yelled through the door.

I used the tools to remove the pins from the door hinges. I had a student at the time, and he made his way into the apartment and used a multi-tool to remove the elbow from the top of the door. With the door removed, the firefighters helped us extricate the man from the rubble. I glanced at the spot he was lying in and saw a flatted out rat he had been on top of for who knows how long!

Carefully and slowly, we took him down the stairs and into the ambulance. It took six of us to do the job safely, and we hurry to the hospital where were received right away. One of the paramedic crews who were already at the hospital gave us a hand transferring the patient over to the hospital bed.

"Is that a toothbrush in his foot?" one of the medics asked.

I looked, and embedded into the skin of his right foot and ankle, was a toothbrush. I found out later that he had been lying in one place so long that the toothbrush burrowed its way into his foot. Miraculously, he made a full medical recovery before being sent off to psych.

Season: Summer
Time: 1930hrs
Weather: Hot, hazy, 30°C
Area Demographic: Run down house, urban core
Dispatch Info: 75yo male, short of breath

It was the kind of hot where you feel sticky all over. My partner and I got to the address and the fire department, a crew I knew well, was already there. They were always willing to help. The house was split into many different apartments, and the one we needed to get to was at the back with a small alleyway that led to it. We entered the small apartment and the wife greeted us. She was sitting on a commode and wheeling herself around.

This is strange.

I listened as she gave me a rundown of the situation. I looked over while listening to her and saw the patient. He was in a hospital bed, naked and almost four hundred pounds. The wife told me he'd been sick all day and couldn't breathe. My partner and I rushed over and started assessing and treating him. He was really ill; the cardiac monitor showed him to be going in and out of ventricular tachycardia (V-tach), a potentially lethal heart arrhythmia. At this point, my attention was entirely focused on the patient. It was a complicated extrication.

The patient demanded to go to the washroom, which was a lengthy process. He sat up with his feet on the floor at the side of the bed, placed a pail between his legs and urinated. His belly was so big that it covered his front and hung between his knees. The urine dripped off his stomach and into the bucket below. To his credit, he wiped himself off thoroughly before coming with us.

As we began extrication, he must have let out a silent but deadly fart, cause it got pretty ripe in there. As we were leaving, I thanked the fire department, and my partner pointed out something that I didn't want to know. He said that the ripe smell wasn't coming from the patient, it was the wife taking a dump right in front of us and the fire crew on the commode. My attention was so focused on the patient that I didn't notice.

No matter where the patient is, I will continue to serve them to the best of my ability. With every less-than-tidy place I visit, it gets easier and less of a shock. I keep in mind the diversity of the human race, the spectrum of cultures and income demographics. It helps me pass less judgement on patients and more treatment.

Chapter song selection:
"We Gotta Get Outta This Place" by The Animals

Chapter 7

The COVID-19 Pandemic

I turned forty in January of 2020. I usually don't celebrate my birthday but forty is a big one, so I invited my friends via Facebook to get together at a bar that had pinball machines and a few arcade games from the 90s like Terminator 2 and Mortal Kombat. People came without masks or hand sanitizer, we drank, hugged and stood next to each other. Little did I know what was coming or that this would be the last time people in Ontario would gather this way for a long time.

    I was about to seek a publisher for this book in February of 2020 when the pandemic hit and turned the world we knew upside down and backwards. Contradictory rules, failed leadership and guidelines that didn't make sense. Never before had I faced so many rapid changes as a paramedic. I'm sure you out there had your share of complaints of how this was handled as well.

I decided that I had to write about my experiences during the pandemic. How could I approach a publisher without including my experiences with the most significant medical challenge that my generation has faced? The pandemic would challenge us in ways I never thought possible. It would cause many of us to leave the job, and it accelerated burnout.

It would also indicate that we learned nothing from the 2003 SARS outbreak. Even back then, PPE went into short supply. Since that virus was not as transmissible, it fizzled out and did not make it into my community. We wore masks back then and started a cleaning routine that had not previously been done or enforced. As you well know, the PPE problem and prevention of transmission would fuel the beginning of the pandemic for months. It would also strike fear and anxiety into me on a level I had not experienced before. Like my coworkers, I hid it well.

As paramedics, we had to wear gowns, masks and safety goggles on almost every call. It was difficult getting used to putting these on before patient contact, especially before someone who was VSA. I was so used to moving quickly to get to the patient, but now I had to put on all this PPE before getting out of the ambulance. For the first while I was pretty anxious and impatient to get to the call while donning the PPE. I was allergic to the first round of surgical masks, and my face broke out in severe eczema that took me a week and a few tubes of hydrocortisone to recover from. I then wore a North 7700 mask for an entire year until N95s were in good supply. I lost my voice a few times because I had to yell most of the time.

These are just a few excerpts from that time we'd all like to forget.

Season: Winter
Time: 1340hrs
Weather: Cold, -14°C
Area Demographic: Suburban townhome
Dispatch Info: 19yo female, COVID-19 positive, short of breath

This call happened when testing was widespread and cases were confirmed. Before there was consistent testing, cases were not confirmed, so we treated most patients as positive cases with a wide array of symptoms. This created an anxiety in me that I spoke of earlier. It was the fear of the unknown and what COULD happen that created the fear. Virtually every call I would think to myself

Am I going to get Covid? Am I going to bring it to my family?

I would concentrate on following proper PPE applications to ensure I had the best chance of keeping the virus at bay. With that in mind on every call since the pandemic hit, my partner and I donned all the PPE and headed into the danger zone.

The woman met us at the door and I could see she was breathing heavily. We got the stretcher as close to the patient as possible and let her get on. Diligently, she had her own personal oxygen monitor on her finger and showed it to us. It read in the low eighties (normal should be about ninety-five to one hundred). Through broken, winded sentences she stumbled out, "That's why I called you guys; I can't breathe." We treated with oxygen right away and got her into the back of the ambulance.

The back of an ambulance is a box that is about five by ten by five feet. Tight quarters when you have a virus in the air and the only thing protecting you is your mask and an exhaust fan that is only five inches wide. This also created anxiety in me during the first couple of waves. In time, I would realize that the mask was the most important piece of PPE. Only after the first six months did I settle down a bit.

We were instructed to withhold many respiratory symptom relief therapies during the pandemic to minimize the danger to us. I think it was a big mistake as this patient qualified for some therapies that we could not give at the time.

Through her medical history we found out that she was involved in a significant cycling accident and had lost her spleen. You can live without your spleen, but your ability to fight infections can be limited as it is a reservoir for blood and makes white blood cells. It was common information at this time that immunocompromised individuals were more susceptible to severe COVID-19 infections, and this was such a case. The patient deteriorated en route, and before we left the hospital she was intubated and on a ventilator.

This was the first case that hit home for me. I had made hundreds of patient contacts at this point in the pandemic, but this was the first confirmed case of

COVID-19 in a young individual that I saw deteriorate before my eyes. I made sure to air out the back, clean it and wash my hands before I removed my mask. Then on to the next one…

Season: Spring
Time: 0800hrs
Weather: Cool, 8°C
Area Demographic: Urban home
Dispatch Info: 30yo male, vital signs absent

This was my first cardiac arrest during the pandemic, and I took time to put on all the PPE. I felt that I was taking away from the patient's chances of survival as this procedure took time. The gown covered the equipment that was on my belt and pockets, so I bought a side bag to keep all my personal paramedic equipment in. We were motioned by police to the garage where the patient was located.

The fire department had started resuscitation and warned us there were needles on the ground. This was an obvious cardiac arrest caused by an overdose. I figured he had died sometime in the early morning and there was little chance for us to bring him back.

There was no electricity in the garage, but the fire department provided a portable light that lit up the entire room brightly. We carefully took over resuscitation from the fire department. It was hard getting used to having a gown on, and my safety goggles fogged up a little, but I got through it. We finished the resuscitation and pronounced him in the garage.

I went to deliver the death notification to his brother, who was letting him stay in the garage because he had nowhere to go. He wouldn't let him in the house because of his habits. I explained to him how many people I had seen die alone on the streets and that giving his brother a place to stay was exemplary. I touched his shoulder and thanked him for doing that, attempting to comfort the man in a tragic moment. Overdose deaths would rise significantly during the pandemic. This was just the beginning.

Season: Winter
Time: 0000hrs
Weather: Cold, -16°C
Area Demographic: Urban home
Dispatch Info: Police requesting ambulance for a domestic

A few weeks into the first lockdown, we noticed that domestic violence calls were on the rise. People were being forced to stay at home with their abuser, which escalated the violence with frequency and intensity. It was one of the many negative by-products of the pandemic. We got no information from the police, so we did not know what we were walking into.

Rolling up on-scene we saw the police talking to a man who was bleeding from his nose. I assumed we were here for him and asked if he was okay. He scoffed at me angrily and told me his injuries were nothing. Then he stepped into the house and pointed out the rampage his girlfriend had gone on.

It looked like a war zone.

I could tell it was a newly-renovated kitchen with a modern look. All but a few cupboards were smashed and there was red wine and broken glass everywhere. The police confirmed that the girlfriend had left and was not on scene. This was always important to confirm as there have been a few times that the assailant hadn't left the scene and things got hairy.

The man then asked me to go to the back of the house to check on his son. There, in a small pool of blood was a fifteen-year-old boy with a laceration on his foot. During the domestic, he had gone to get the cat out of the fray and stepped on some of the broken glass and cut his foot pretty good. I was surprised at his calm demeanour considering what he had just been through. We bandaged him up and took him to the hospital. His sister wanted to come along and we let her. During the ride to the hospital, they made light of the situation by making jokes about the new kitchen. They got on their phones and made arrangements with friends to stay the night somewhere else. I made small talk about what they wanted to do after high school. They both had plans to go to a university away from home. I was impressed and admired their attitude towards their situation. It was a courage against adversity that I hoped my daughters could have someday. But I'm going to do the best job I can as a father and husband so that their chance to showcase courage won't come from a situation like that.

COME RIDE WITH ME

Season: Spring
Weather: Cool and clear
Area Demographic: Suburban apartment building
Dispatch info: Imminent labour

My partner and I had never delivered a baby even though we had more than thirty-five years of experience between us at that point in time. I had come within seconds of many deliveries, getting there just to see the baby already in mothers' arms, but I had never been there to witness that first cry of a brand-new life. Having a baby is stressful enough and the pandemic must have compounded the stress.

Masks, gowns and gloves on, we entered the apartment to the cries of a woman in labour. Our initial assessment of the apartment and family indicated this was a Middle Eastern household. That night I was working with Sarah Batchelor, one of the best advanced care paramedic students I'd had the pleasure of teaching, so it was more culturally sensitive for her to do the hands-on delivery. She was already a nurse, so she had more experience than I did at this sort of thing anyway.

We made our way to the bedroom. The woman was already on the floor and we saw the head of the baby coming out. I stood by with obstetrics equipment while Sarah successfully delivered the baby. Within a few seconds the room was filled with the first cries of a new life. A smile broke out on all of our faces, and the new bouncing baby boy was healthy. Once the husband knew that the baby was healthy, he promptly asked James and I to leave the room. We respected their culture and exited with haste.

That morning, James and I had a coffee together to celebrate finally having delivered a baby. The sun was just coming over the horizon, and the sky was golden. Healthy babies are one of the only real happy calls paramedics go on. This happened a week before my twentieth year, and it was nice to have finally delivered a baby.

Season: Winter
Time: 1940
Weather: Cold, no precipitation, -14°C
Area Demographic: Nursing home
Dispatch Info: Palliative, COVID-19 positive

I was told that the patient had tested positive for the omicron variant three days prior and was now palliative. Her oxygen saturations were in the low eighties, and her respiratory rate was over forty. By this time in the pandemic, we knew when the end was near for COVID-19 patients, and this woman was at the point of no return. Her roommate had tested positive a few days earlier, and it was only a matter of time until the omicron strain made its way to her as well.

Except this wasn't a patient. It was my aunt.

When I was twenty-two, I signed up to be executor to my aunt and uncle. When my uncle passed away, he left behind a wife suffering from dementia. They had no other family that could help. I helped get her into a great nursing home that gave her exemplary care over the next several years. During the last few, the progression of dementia slowly but surely ripped away her quality of life. If you haven't seen this before, you haven't had enough life experience. My daughter would play violin and I strummed the guitar through video conferencing during the pandemic when we couldn't physically go up to see her. It was one of the only things I could do to enrich her life near the end.

Now the end was near, and I went to visit her for the last time. As if I were a paramedic, I put on my Honeywell N7700 with p100 filters, a face shield, gown and gloves. As I entered the room, I could tell she was close to passing. She was breathing rapidly and only responsive to pain. I told her that she was loved and that she should go see her husband Andy, and Bobbie, my mother and her best friend who had left us a couple of years before.

I was hesitant about staying with her until the end because I had young girls at home, a job and a wife to take care of. These things weighed on me but, sadly, I said my goodbye and left her to die alone in that room.

I'll feel guilty until the day I die, but if there is anything that makes me feel better, it's the fact that I was there when she lived, and I enriched her life when I could. It's the time we spend with the living that will matter most when a person is not with us anymore.

Season: Fall
Time: 1230hrs
Weather: Cool, overcast, 14°C
Area Demographic: Highway overpass
Dispatch Info: Unconscious male in mental distress

As the call details came through, I was confused on how dispatch knew that the man was in mental distress when he was unconscious as well. I thought maybe he was having a mental health crisis, then went unconscious—or vice versa. We were on the way to the call when I spotted a man running towards us on the sidewalk with another man not far behind chasing him. I only saw the man for a split second as he approached us, but he looked determined and desperate. I knew this was our patient, so I asked our new recruit to stop the ambulance as I opened the door.

"I WANNA DIE!" he screamed at the top of his lungs.

We are on an overpass for a 100km/h highway. He's gonna jump off this bridge!

Without thinking, I leapt from the ambulance and started chasing him. I didn't put my gown and safety goggles on like I was supposed to, but I had a mask on. He looked back at me and realized I was gaining on him. Not that I practice sprinting, but I do keep in decent shape and can run pretty fast for a man in his forties. But the mask made it difficult to breathe, and I started panting. The man cut to the edge of the bridge and began climbing over as I caught up. As he was letting go with his upper body and hands, I pinned one of his legs to the bar with my hands and torso. I made a lightning-quick decision NOT to put my chest over the bar, no matter what the outcome. My weight would have carried over the railing, putting me at significantly more risk of plummeting off the bridge with him. This was my limit I set to help this man.

With his leg pinned to the bar, I could hold him there for a while. Within a few seconds, my partner and the bystander who was chasing him caught up with me.

"K guys, don't put your chest over the bar, keep on this side!" I directed. "When I say go, we will all reach over, grab him with one hand each and pull him over. Ready? GO!"

It worked! But no good deed goes unpunished. He got up and started fighting us to get back over the bridge. Thinking of George Floyd and not wanting to hurt him, I engaged the patient in a hand-to-hand confrontation, taking care not to injure him. He tried to punch me, but more than thirty years of martial arts training kicked in and I blocked his incoming attack. I got a solid hold of both of his arms and gently foot swept him to the ground. At this point he was face up with his back on the roadway as the fight had spilled out onto the street.

I then took a basic Brazilian jiu-jitsu position called high mount, which means I sat high on his chest with my knees up in his armpits. He couldn't get up but tried to punch and bite me. As I radioed for help, he knocked the device out of my hand, so my partner went back to the main radio in the ambulance and called for backup.

All this happened so fast—less than two minutes in real time. My opponent —er, patient—realized that he would not win the battle and uttered something I will never forget.

"Fuck you Liu Kang!" he yelled.

For those of you who don't know, Liu Kang is a character in the video game Mortal Kombat. He can shoot fireballs out of his hands and has a devastating flying kick. It was funny because I never hurt patients in scuffles. It takes a tremendous amount of restraint and skill to be able to subdue a mentally ill patient without hurting them. A skill not many people have.

My partner returned and let me know help was on the way. I looked up to see that cars had stopped and were probably filming at this point. Out of breath now, I could hear the sirens of the police. Two more ambulances arrived with a few police units. Everybody grabbed a limb and we all lifted the patient onto the stretcher and I sedated him.

At the hospital, the adrenaline dump happened and I went a little pale for a moment while giving a report to the triage nurse. The nurse got me some juice and I continued my handover report. During this, I told the doc about the Brazilian jiu-jitsu high mount.

"I'm gonna try that on my wife tonight," he said with a coy smile.

The staff cracked up too.

Two years later, I would be a recipient of the first Ontario Medal for Paramedic Bravery for this act. It was a prestigious night in Queen's Park at the legislative assembly of Ontario. The pandemic had been declared over, gatherings were in full swing without masks, and I put on my dress uniform for the first time other than for a funeral. I took a moment when I put it on to dwell on the idea that this was going to be a celebration rather than a remembrance.

Nine of us received the award that night. While talking to the other paramedics, I realized I was in the presence of greatness. One woman dove down fifteen feet to rescue a man from the bottom of a lake. Another pair of medics overturned an aircraft with help and extricated the patients. All the stories were above and beyond the call of duty for a paramedic, and we were all humbled by the event.

Our citations about our feats were read as we were presented our medals by the Lieutenant Governor of Ontario and the Minister of Health. Then, a dinner fit for a wedding was held at the Royal Ontario Museum. The Queen's Own's Rifles played music in the background as we enjoyed a wonderful meal. It was an experience that I'll remember forever. I felt so lucky to have received the medal and that everything worked out on a positive note.

Because every paramedic has been present when things turn out negative.

I thought of a scene from *Karate Kid Part II* when Mr. Miyagi was telling Daniel about his medal of honour.

"Dis say you brave," Mr. Miyagi says, patting Daniel-san's chest with an open hand where his heart is. "Dis say you lucky," he said, pointing to the medal.

I didn't understand that in 1986.

I don't know if I'll make another patient contact without a mask now that the COVID-19 pandemic has passed. Due to diligent PPE donning and doffing, I seemed to dodge the bullet, even though I was in and around patients and hospitals riddled with the disease. Unfortunately, one of my kids brought it home asymptomatically. My family survived and we were glad for things to get back to normal. Let's hope it stays that way ... and we can be thankful for what we have.

For the happiest of people don't have what they want. They want what they already have.

Chapter song selection:
"Mad World" by Gary Jules

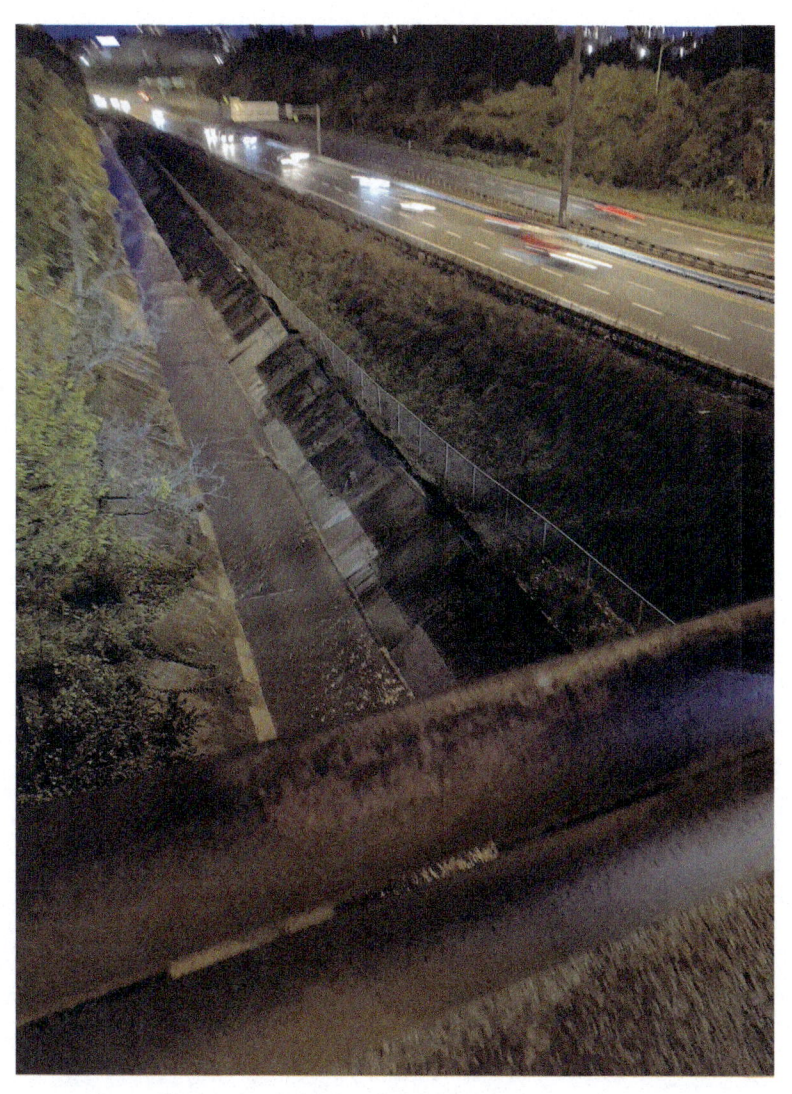

The railing where I pinned the man's leg, stopping him from falling

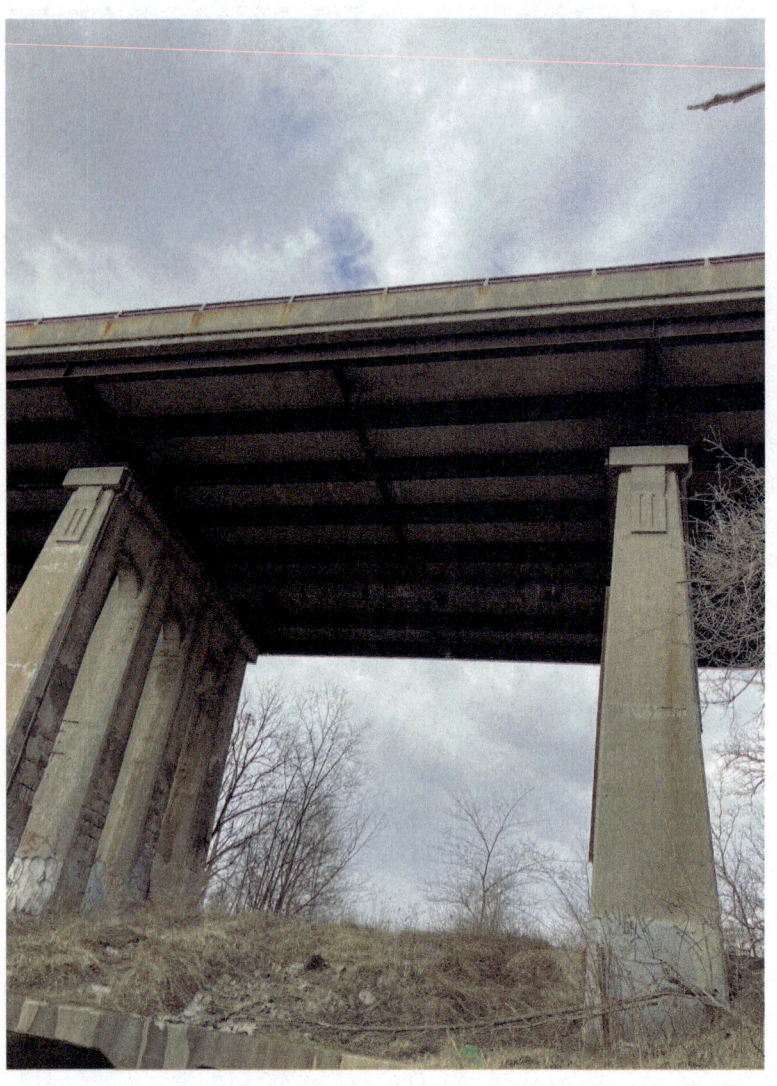

The view from below that bridge

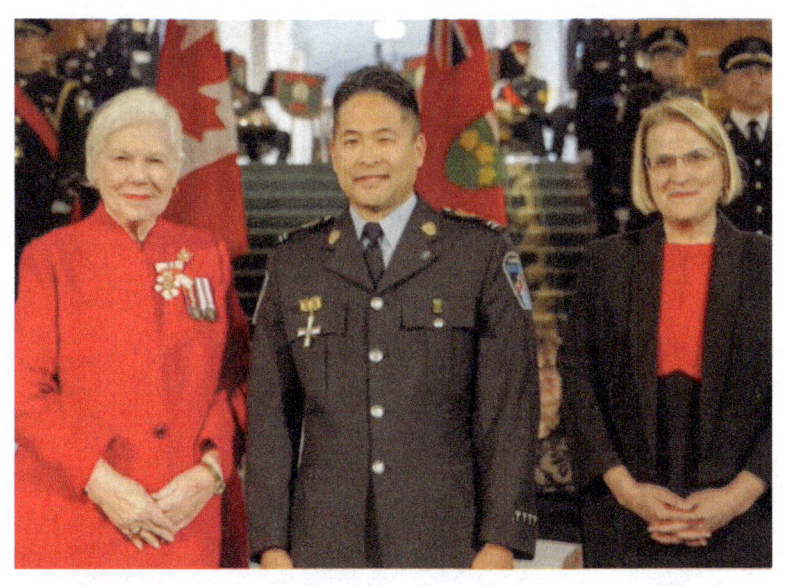

Receiving the medal from
Lieutenant Governor Elizabeth Dowdeswell
and Minister of Health Sylvia Jones

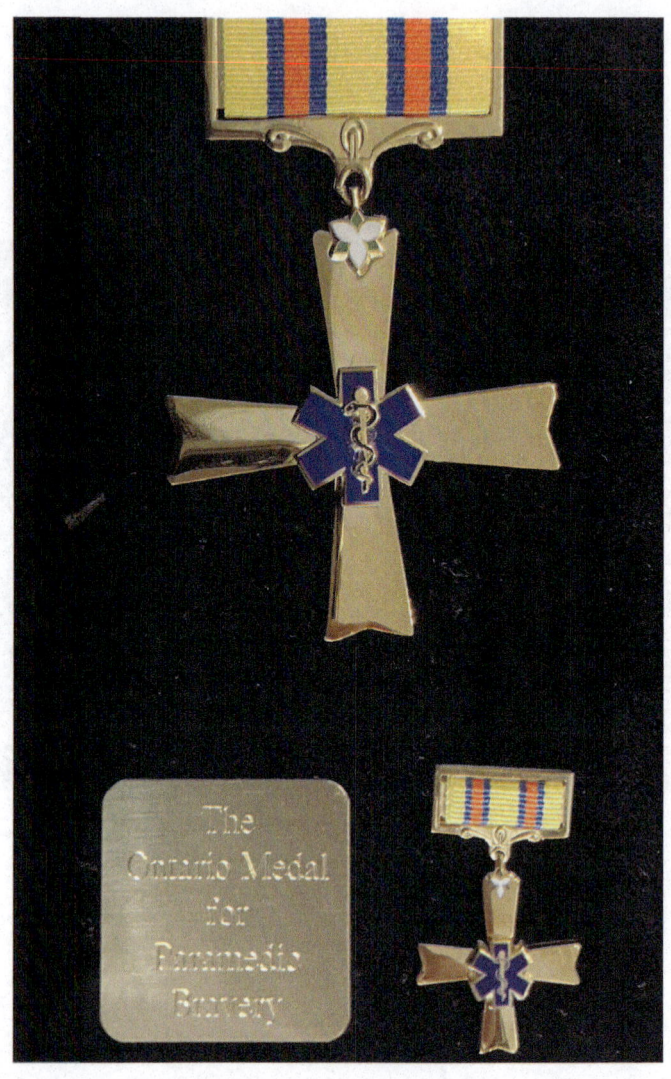

The inaugural Ontario Medal
for Paramedic Bravery.

Chapter 8

Remarkable People

As I have mentioned, Hamilton has provided a dynamic and diverse experience as a paramedic. In a typical shift, I transport an average of seven patients, which equates to about one thousand patients in a year. In my most active year so far, I made over 1200 patient contacts (I worked a lot of overtime shifts that year!). The volume of exposure means I encounter many different characters and personalities. One moment I could be picking up a homeless person from an alleyway and the next call could bring me to the doorstep of a three-storey mansion or to the woods during a downpour. This was one of the things that attracted me to the job. The ever-changing atmosphere creates possibilities to meet an endless number of diverse people.

Season: Winter
Time: 0400hrs
Weather: Clear, cold, -10°C
Area Demographic: Gated seniors' community
Dispatch Info: 87yo male, uncontrolled bleed

This man decided to get a glass of water at four o'clock in the morning. He dropped it and stepped on a shard of glass, causing a laceration on the bottom of his foot. The blood thinners he was on made a huge puddle of blood on the kitchen floor. My partner cleaned it up while I took the piece of glass out of his foot and assessed the wound. It was minor and would not require stitches. The good news for him was he would get to stay in the comfort of his home. I bandaged his foot up, and we started our paperwork.

He began chatting up a storm. His voice was full of enthusiasm as he told us he served in World War II as an intelligence officer. By the end of the war, he had achieved the rank of Command Sergeant Major, a high rank. When Germany surrendered, one of their highest-ranking intelligence officers did not want to surrender to a low-ranking officer. Apparently, most of the high-ranking officers were off celebrating at the time and the German officer considered Command Sergeant Major to be a worthy rank, so he formally surrendered to our patient.

"What was that moment like?" I asked, intrigued.

He paused for a second, relaxed and replied, "We both looked at each other with relief that the war was finally over."

After that, he led us to his room that had a wall with medals and newspaper articles on it. The most striking piece was a commendation from George S. Patton.

As he probably wouldn't need stitches, we left him in the comfort of his home, thanked him for his stories and returned to base.

I always feel privileged to meet veterans of the Second World War and I thought to myself right there that they would all be gone someday. This call happened in the early 2000s when many WWII veterans were still around. Today, there are few, if any, left. Tomorrow there will be none. That's why November 11 is an important day for me.

A few years later, I picked him up again for shortness of breath. He had moved to the nursing home in the same community and his wife had passed away. The nurses all loved him and told us that he was a smooth talker. So much so that he had two girlfriends on the go—at ninety years of age.

Season: Winter
Time: 0445hrs
Weather: Cool, no snow on the ground
Area Demographic: Residential urban
Dispatch info: 20yo, vital signs absent

Twenty-year-old men don't go into cardiac arrest very often. Usually, it is due to trauma or a drug overdose. This call happened the year that the opioid crisis started. Management ran a briefing on this, but we didn't believe it until it started becoming a routine call. There was a potent batch of fentanyl going around during this time, and I assumed this was the cause of the cardiac arrest. Then I got an update from dispatch.

"Patient has a condition called *pro-gear-ia*?" There was confusion in the dispatcher's voice.

"What is that?" James asked.

I took a deep breath and keyed the mic, "That's pronounced progeria; it's an advanced aging disease, extremely rare. We're in uncharted territory."

Before I wanted to become a paramedic, I already had interest in the medical field. I watched *E.R.*, *Scrubs* and any medical documentary that was aired on cable (yes, cable television on a cathode ray screen!). One documentary I watched was on these special people. Progeria is a genetic disease that causes patients to age rapidly; they are often small with elderly faces. Average life expectancy is fourteen years, and it's not uncommon for strokes and heart attacks to hit them before their tenth birthday.

This was all running through my head when we were going to the call.

I opened the door and saw something beautiful … timeless love. Sitting on the couch was a mother I estimated to be in her late thirties. In her lap was her beloved son, life leaving him too early, barely breathing. She was looking into his eyes and gently caressing his bald head. She knew what was happening and would have known their time was limited from the day of his diagnosis. Even though no words were coming out of her mouth, I knew she was saying goodbye. I could see she had been a courageous mother, devoting her life to making the most of their time together. She had lived her life for him and now it was coming to an end. This was one of the most beautiful things I have ever witnessed.

I approached the mother at her side and gave her an extra moment with her son.

"Ma'am, we're going to try and help your son," I said in the softest, kindest voice I could.

She looked away with sadness in her eyes and gave him up for the last time. I started what I knew would be a futile resuscitation.

This was one of the most challenging calls of my career. We were dealing with one of the rarest and most unique conditions (I would find out later this was one of three patients in Canada), and we had seconds to decide about treatment. Keeping in mind that these people are petite, I estimated this patient to be about sixty-five pounds and three feet tall, adult settings and pads for the defibrillator wouldn't make sense, neither would adult drug settings. I decided to use pediatric defibrillator pads and drug doses. He still had a pulse as we laid him on the floor. Blood was coming up his airway, so I thought I'd suction and intubate right away. His anatomy was different from adults and pediatrics. I got one look with my laryngoscope and knew I would have trouble.

James tapped me on the shoulder. He looked at me with concern and guidance.

"We should go," he said.

James was one of the best partners I've ever had. In that one sentence he communicated that he could see I was going to have trouble. That this call was beyond our scope. There were going to be delays in treatment and transport because I was probably going to get focused on a skill like an IV. It was better to get moving while we could. These are the marks of a great partner.

So I listened.

We loaded him up and sped to the hospital as his heart beat for the last time. Despite IV epinephrine and all efforts, we couldn't get his heart started again. I patched to the hospital to be ready for us. When we arrived, I gave a report as the hospital staff began their resuscitation protocols.

After I had finished handing off care, I hastily went to the washroom and cried at work for the first time in fifteen years. The combination of the picture I saw when I walked in the house, coupled with what I knew, got me thinking how lucky I am to have my healthy daughter at home.

It hit me all at once.

I let it all out for a couple of minutes, pulled myself together, waited till the red eyes were gone and got ready for the next call. The mother was in the quiet room—the place they put you in to give you bad news. She was alone, and I decided to have the bad news conversation with her.

"I want to thank you for what you did for my son," was the first thing she said.

It took me by surprise.

"I'm so proud of him, he accomplished so much," she added.

I led her back to talk to the doctor to stop resuscitation, and she said goodbye for the last time.

What I perceived when I walked into the house for the first time couldn't have been more accurate. I found out through a co-worker that she had indeed done everything she could for her son. She had been on *The Maury Povich Show* so her son could meet his favourite band NSYNC at the age of four. He was an exceptional Ti-Cat fan, and the team took him in as one of their own. He attended many of their games, and his house held the Grey Cup for a time. He also had an honorary pilot's licence. This man had accomplished more in his twenty years than most, all due to his mother's diligence. Thanks to his mother. I didn't know anything about Devin Scullion before this call, but I did after I saw timeless love in his house.

Season: Summer
Time: 1434hrs
Weather: Warm, 20°C
Area Demographic: Industrial complex
Dispatch Info: Industrial accident

We didn't get much information from dispatch on this call, but they assured us that we knew everything they did. The caller was hesitant to convey information and we would soon find out why.

As we approached a large industrial building, I wondered what they made. My gut feeling suggested I should get my safety helmet just in case. I put it on, and a man in a dress shirt and slacks, a supervisor of some kind, met us at the doorway.

Without making eye contact he said, "Um, you're here for a boy. It's bad."

"What happened?"

My questions were cut short as he walked towards the scene of the accident and made a hasty exit. I came to realize that people have different reactions to emergencies.

I could tell this man was very concerned, and his way of dealing with it was keeping his mouth shut. It could have also been because this could prove to be a preventable workplace accident.

But it is not my place to judge, and we would have more important things to take care of in a few seconds.

My partner and I entered and saw a sixteen-year-old boy lying on his back on the ground. His left arm had an open humerus fracture, his legs were motionless, and his right leg was bent back underneath him so much so that his foot was sticking out from the top of his head like a periscope. Above him was the most gargantuan piece of steel I have ever seen. It was approximately five feet tall, eight feet wide and six inches thick. I would later find out that it was half a door to a nuclear reactor. It weighed ten tonnes. I also noticed that nobody was by the boy's side. I only had seconds to process this scene, but it bothered me to no end later that in this person's time of need, nobody in that building cared enough to come to his side.

The massive piece of steel was tilted over, but being held up by a crane and men were scrambling to support it. I noticed that nobody was wearing a hard hat. *Do we wait for the fire department and workers to make things safe? Or do we just go and get the patient?* My partner and I concluded that there was no time to waste, and we didn't have confidence in the staff there.

Despite the area not being safe, we dragged the patient out from underneath the ten-tonne door. I remember looking up at it and thinking that my death would be swift if it fell again.

From the time we met the man outside the door to this moment was less than a minute.

Now that we were somewhat safe, I said, "Hey man! What's your name?"

"Eric. Can you please give me something to put me to sleep so I can wake up fixed?" he asked.

Knowing I could not do this, I replied, "I'm going to treat you like you were my own brother. I'm going to take care of you the best I can."

With that, we expedited to the hospital. I peered out the window from the back of the ambulance and saw that the police had blocked intersections for us to clear a path to the hospital. We made it in record time.

Two days later I visited Eric in the hospital. He was all casted up and told me what happened. It's a familiar story that should not be told more than once. Eric was a co-op student that was asked to do something unsafe. Not wanting to disappoint, he went and did it anyway, and it almost cost him his life. Open fractured humerus, fractured pelvis, bilateral femur fractures, and tibia-fibula fracture was the short list of injuries he sustained. That doesn't include the soft tissue injuries that occurred as well. I wondered if he would walk again.

Months later, Eric wanted to meet us and thank us for saving his life. My partner and I were humbled as the young man approached us and stood before us with a smile. A cane supported him and he had an uncontrollable leg tremor. I couldn't believe it, but he walked towards us and shook our hands.

"I'm gonna be a paramedic," Eric said with confidence.

"We'll do everything we can to make that happen," I said.

My partner and I shoot each other an unresolved look. We both knew of the physical demands of the job and remained doubtful.

A few years later, I celebrated with Eric as he passed his provincial paramedic exam. I had been his preceptor and had trained him in the field. Eric has truly amazed and humbled me in many ways, and I have never been so happy to be proven wrong.

Meeting diverse people in times of crisis is a privilege that I appreciate every shift. I look forward to the people I will meet in the future, and the ever-changing assortment of personalities and histories I will bear witness to.

Chapter Song selection:
"You're Beautiful" by James Blunt

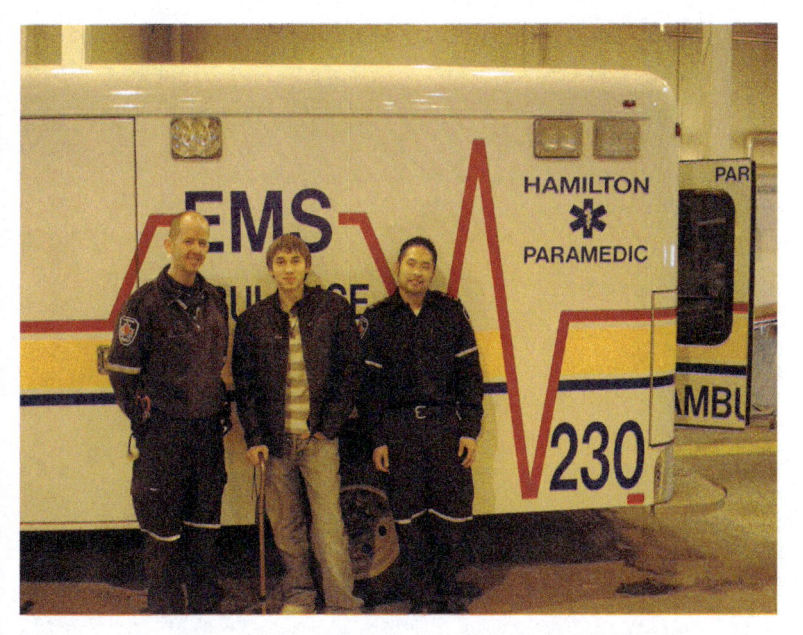

Eric coming to thank us for his eventful day

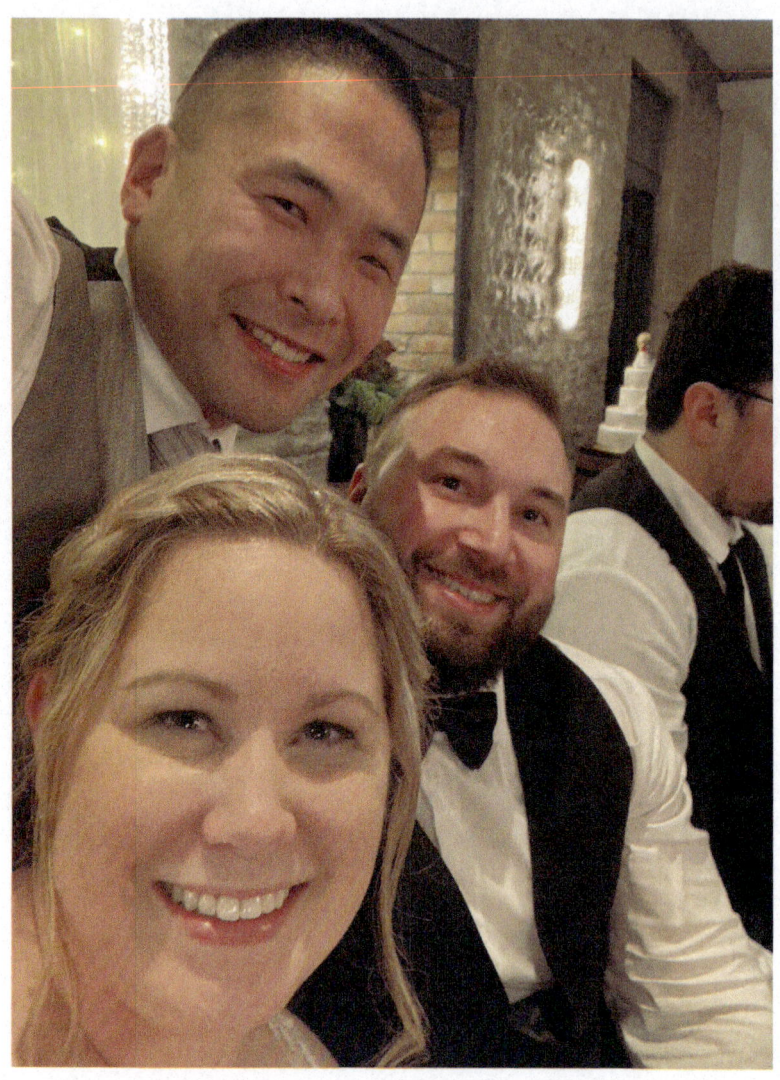

Eric many years later on his wedding day. I'm privileged to still be in his life. The challenges he has overcome have made him my personal hero.

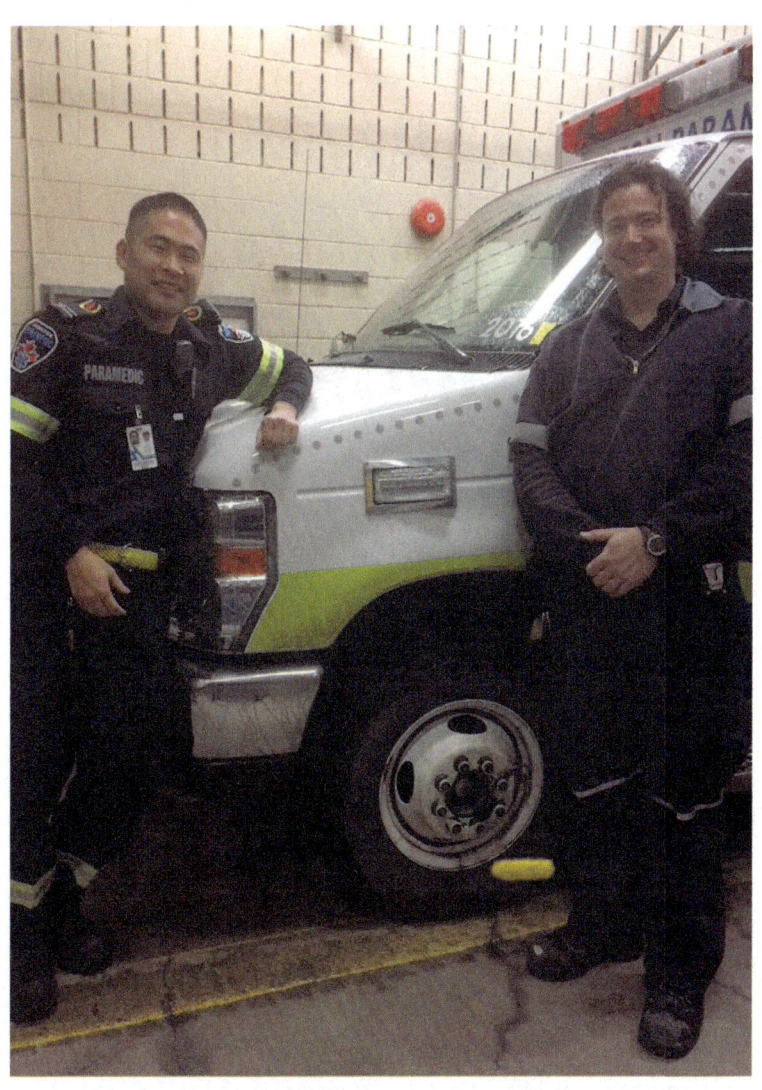

One of my best partners, James Watson, and I in 2016. We made 1200 patient contacts that year with 49 of them vital signs absent.

Chapter 9

Frequent Flyers

Every frequent flyer we meet has a history of mental illness. We know their medical history, birth dates and addresses by heart. Sometimes, even just the way the call is dispatched will tip us off that it is a patient we know. Most of these patients are on social assistance, so they never have to pay for the ambulance. Consequently, it is not uncommon for them to call eight times a week.

Yes, that is more than one time a day.

One particular patient called forty times in one month! Due to legality issues and liability, we can never deny them care.

There are times when their complaints are legitimate. Working for more than twenty years, the potential to see these patients at their moment of death or a real medical emergency is high. So no matter how many times I came in contact with these patients, I kept the aforementioned in my back pocket.

Well, most of the time.

I'm not perfect, and I speak for most paramedics when I say that I can and do run out of patience. When you see a system fail and patients not getting the help they need, paramedics can lose empathy for them. They become short and stern with these individuals. Sometimes this induces an argument and escalates to violence. Many paramedics say frequent flyers are one of the leading causes of burnout.

One paramedic had a quote that helped me treat these patients with respect. This medic was the definition of professional. He was fit and trim at over sixty years of age, and there always was a polished shine to his shoes and a tie on his shirt. He also rocked a handlebar moustache. Jimmy Masterton was his name. In his infinite wisdom, he would ask young medics what the definition of an emergency was. Many people would reply with gunshot wounds or a heart attack. Jimmy would respond, "When a person finds themselves in a situation they cannot handle themselves."

I kept this in mind when I met up with frequent flyers.

Fortunately, I met this paramedic when I was a student, and I have never burned out. I still have to remind myself to treat these patients like it was the first time even when I've met them twice in the same shift (yes that does happen!). Names, circumstances and details have been changed to protect identities.

Season: All of them
Time: Anytime
Weather: All weather
Area Demographic: Messy apartment or the street
Dispatch Info: Male, intoxicated, for a fall

Dave Books had been calling us for more than a decade. He was in his thirties, tall and slender, with long hair. The call was usually dispatched for a fall. We always went, picked him up off the floor and took him to the hospital. Sometimes he didn't want to go, so we left him there. That was usually followed up by more drinking, falling and calling.

His messy apartment was always littered with empty alcohol bottles of every sort. Last time, I counted at least ten twenty-four-hour AA sober coins, which meant he had made an effort to get better. But many of the medics looked at him as a disgrace and failure. A complete waste of time.

Keeping in mind what Jimmy Masterton's definition of an emergency is, I always treated him with respect and empathy. I never had a problem with him. But a few years ago, he had fallen and broken a vessel in his brain. This led to a cerebral bleed that left him with permanent brain damage. Since then, he became increasingly aggressive and it was hard to keep him calm. Our medics lost patience with him pretty fast, and I have to continually remind myself to be patient. I don't know what drove this man to the bottle, and I am thankful I'm not in his position.

One day I stood behind him in line at the liquor store (I was off duty!), and watched him buy his fix. This was one of the few times I had seen him sober.

Alcohol is an overlooked problem. I remember attending assemblies and presentations on the subject in high school. I thought it was overkill because I was young and naive. Even before I became a paramedic, I knew people that drank too much before they drove. Later on, I would have friends that had problems with the substance. The good things are that there are many programs to help and the stigma around alcoholism is not as strong as it once was.

Season: All of them
Time: Anytime
Weather: All weather
Area Demographic: On the streets or in his apartment
Dispatch Info: Failure to cope or suicidal ideations

Kyle Lars, another patient I'd picked up for over a decade, was the definition of a lost soul. He stood almost six feet and had long hair. There wasn't a mental health diagnosis he hadn't had, his medications were changed many times, and his outer forearms were almost entirely covered with cutting scars.

His call always came in as a suicidal male. When we got to him, he was usually booming with energy, pacing around and yelling. I'd heard he can get quite violent. Like Dave Books, I treated him with respect and empathy, and he was never aggressive with me. I found that tone of voice and showing a little care can go a long way with him. I ran into Kyle many times while not on a call but on duty. He was usually already at the hospital or on the streets. I found him to be extraordinarily chatty and occasionally cheerful during these times.

I respected Kyle for his living space. He did not have much, but he took care of what he had. When we went to his place, it was always as clean as a whistle. I found it amazing that a person with such a disorganized personality could find such organization in cleanliness.

One time, I sliced my hand trying to catch a glass that fell off the counter. It hit the granite top at the same time as I squeezed it. The glass was a thin one and shattered in my hand. I got eight stitches and saw Kyle with another crew at the hospital. He expressed the utmost concern about my cut on my hand, told me to be careful and scolded me for being at work. It was nice to see a patient that cared for the paramedic for once.

Season: All of them
Time: When his caregiver finds her
Weather: All weather
Area Demographic: Residential house
Dispatch Info: Unconscious diabetic

One of our most astounding and notorious patients was a woman I will call Sandy Brown. Sandy was slim, in her fifties and the most brutal diabetic any of us had met.

Here is how the events would happen. Sandy's blood sugar would go low, and she would become unconscious.

Sandy lived with a family member, and when they found her, they would call 911. We would wake her with either a drug called glucagon or inject sugar into her veins. She never wanted to go to the hospital. Sometimes the police would get involved, but she knew what to say to be able to stay home. This would happen up to five times a week, sometimes twice in the same day.

You are probably thinking, *How can this woman do this and not die?* The whole medical community wondered the same. The thing that saved her was the family member who came to her rescue every time. Once they died, we knew it was only a matter of time until she was found dead. We picked her up many times in between the time her family member died and her actual death. One time her blood sugar was high instead of low—almost ten times the normal limit. She was in the hospital for a few weeks and came back home. With her family member not there to save her, soon Sandy was dead.

You get to know these patients after responding to them for over a decade. I discovered that she was a phenomenal cello player and had played in orchestras. Apparently, whenever an orchestra needed a backup cellist, Sandy was the woman to call. She even played for me once. It was phenomenal.

But there was a tragic turning point in Sandy's life that spiraled her downwards: the loss of her child. I never asked what happened or what her child's name was. I saw a single picture of her and her child that looked over a decade old judging by the age of Sandy in the pic. Having children of my own now, I'm glad I treated her with dignity and respect until the end. I don't want to entertain a loss of that magnitude. It pains me to even think of it. Sandy lived it. For that reason, I hope she is reunited with her child.

Season: All
Time: Usually at night
Weather: All types
Area: Subsidized apartments
Dispatch info: Usually an overdose

Amanda and Brady had a tumultuous relationship. They would get into a fight and Brady would get too drunk or overdose on some medication.

In the beginning, Brady could get quite violent. He had a black belt in Tae Kwon Do, so he could be pretty dangerous when he wanted to be. He was tall and robust, so when he didn't want to move, it was tough to make him. Amanda was tall and slender. Brady could get downright nasty and violent at times. But of course, never with me. I used my charm and we kind of bonded over our love for the martial arts. We would converse about our favourite techniques, except for the handful of times he was unresponsive. Amanda went to the hospital with Brady most of the time and was very supportive. I never saw her yell or get upset. I always told Brady that he had an excellent partner—even the police thought that she was a saint.

I found out later that Brady died in some type of tragic accident. I felt for Amanda because, despite how many problems Brady had, she stood by him and loved him. As a paramedic, you venture into the lives and dramas that most of the population binge watch series to capture. I often reflect on these experiences to better my own relationships and remember to be thankful for what I have.

Season: All
Weather: All
Time: Usually during the day
Area: Subsidized apartment
Dispatch info: Female lift assist

The lift assist is something we do all the time. We come pick people up off the floor so they can get on with their day.

Our next frequent flyer used to fall quite a bit. She was a female who had an acquired brain injury at a young age that left her with a multitude of disabilities. She used a wheelchair and had slurred speech. She always had a smile on her face and was very pleasant to us, so my partner and I didn't mind going to pick her up off the floor.

Although she couldn't speak well, she could write like the wind. I read her journal entries every time we went there (with permission, of course), and they expressed the emotions and frustrations she felt about how she could think and feel but couldn't communicate with the world around her. Most of all, she wrote about how impatient and judgemental the world around her was.

She had a few newspaper articles on her walls about her daughter that had been taken into adoption when she was declared unfit to take care of her. There was a picture of her with her daughter who was about one. I learned that she was fighting the courts to make contact with her daughter for many years. This was a dismal situation and I hoped she would get her to wish.

In truly dramatic fashion, she would. When this woman was diagnosed with terminal breast cancer, her family increased the efforts to find her daughter. Meticulously analyzing documents throughout the years, they discovered her daughter's legal name at birth that was overlooked. This led to them finding each other. A reunion was scheduled and the two met again after twenty-four years. It was beautiful to find out that her perseverance paid off. Although she passed only months after finding her daughter, her lifelong dream was fulfilled. The article was published in the local newspaper.

There is a medic superstition that is almost fact when it comes to these patients: When one dies, another pops up. Throughout the years I would see this play out many times. The paramedic social media feed is fast when it comes to the death of a regular and the birth of another. My goal is to stick to the formula of being nice, and I hope it will carry me through to the end of my career.

Chapter song selection:
"Patience", by Guns and Roses

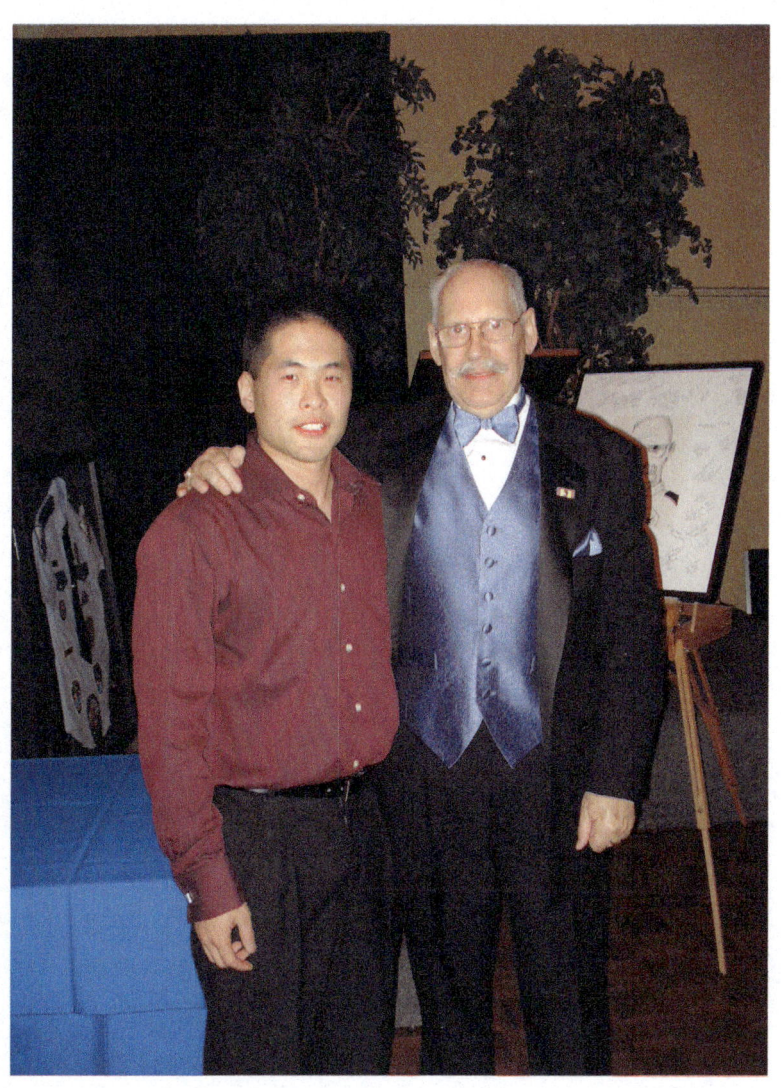

Me with Jimmy Masterton on his retirement day. He was a mentor and the definition of professional paramedic.

Chapter 10

Shots Fired!

The words ring out on the radio. The police will be there in a flash and the intensity kicks up a notch. Paramedics have to be on their game because seconds count.

The region has roughly ten to fifteen gunshot wounds a year, so the chances of being dispatched to one are low. These calls require increased diligence, especially when they are as critical as penetrating trauma is.

There is a push to get off the scene as soon as possible. We treat what we can but get moving to the trauma centre quickly. These calls are high energy and fast paced. Scene times should be under eight minutes. The ride to the hospital is usually crowded because there are police and an extra set of hands in the back. These are the calls we hardcore medics live for.

Season: Fall
Weather: Cool, 10°C
Time: 1700hrs
Area Demographic: Subsidized housing
Dispatch Info: Male shot fifteen times

My partner and I were approaching base when we saw two police cruisers fly by, lights flashing and sirens blaring on the street perpendicular to us. Police typically do not rush to calls unless it is something serious. As we backed into the base, dispatch called us on the radio.

"2067, you're going to a male shot fifteen times."

Fifteen times? That would be a magazine dump if the shots were right in a row without a reload, I thought. *Civilian handguns can only have ten cartridges in the magazine, which could only mean the gun was illegal or a service weapon.*

It was close to shift change and I knew if this turned out to be serious, I wouldn't be home until late. As we blazed through the streets, my partner and I discussed why someone would shoot a person fifteen times. One reason came to mind: domestic dispute gone bad.

Domestics can bring about abnormal scales of violence. Even gang executions are just a few shots at the most. Of course, this was all speculation, and wouldn't change treatment. My mind raced as we approached the scene.

The victim was on the porch on his back and police had already started CPR. We counted one gunshot wound in the chest, three in the abdomen, four in the arms, two in the legs and two in his head. It was dark, and there was little light, so I asked if anyone could see cranial contents (which would mean we could terminate resuscitation). There was none.

I thought we should terminate resuscitation, but the cardiac monitor had a rhythm, a contraindication for termination of resuscitation (TOR) in the field. He was also in view of the public, another reason for us to transport.

We rapidly ushered him into the ambulance, and that's when the blood and cranial contents started gushing out his ears with every compression of CPR. I wish it would have happened on the front porch because I could have stopped. I called a doc to terminate resuscitation because this was going to be messy and futile if we went on. I got the order to terminate and breathed a sigh of relief.

In the province of Ontario, pronouncing somebody in the back of your ambulance makes it a crime scene. We sat in the back with the body for four hours before the coroner instructed us to take the body to the morgue.

The smell of death lingers in the air in that place. Bodies awaiting funerals or autopsies are stacked up and in human size drawers.

The forensics officer told us that he and the detectives always asked themselves, "Will this hold up in court? What do I have to do before I make my next step in the investigation? How can I prove this? Is this obtained by legal means?" For these reasons, they take their time and are 100% focused all the time. James and I watched him put the patient in a body bag and photograph the hands for the pathologist. If he defended himself, there might be skin cells of the murderer underneath his fingernails.

The forensics officer also had to take a picture of himself putting the key into the wall body storage unit to prove it was the right slot for the right body.

Then the coroner showed up.

She was one of the emergency docs that I knew well. She asked a few questions and took pictures of the gunshot wounds. It had been almost six hours since the incident, and the gunshot wounds had visibly changed. The two that were ten centimetres apart on his outside forearm were joined by a line of bruising, which meant that it was one bullet that created an entry and exit wound. The same went for the two holes on his abdomen. They were only three centimetres apart and were also joined by a line of bruising. That could mean he had put his hands up to defend himself and tossed and turned to try to avoid being shot. A desperate measure, futile at point blank range when facing an enraged perpetrator.

The coroner asked us to help slide the body into the wall drawer. I found this quite amusing, as it is something we don't do as paramedics. The last thing she asked me to do was run my gloved finger in the groove of my stretcher mattress to look for shell casings. The groove had blood pooled about one centimetre thick. It was one of the most gruesome things I'd ever done, and I didn't find any casings, so I finally got to go home.

I cycled into work that day, which took fifty minutes. I had been up since four and finally hit the sack at 11:30 p.m. Beat tired, I fell asleep quickly. There is no better sleep medication than sleep deprivation.

Season: Summer
Time: 1830hrs
Weather: Clear and hot, 30°C
Area Demographic: Suburban house
Dispatch Info: Multiple patients with gunshot wounds

It was a student's last day and we carpooled to work. During the ride, one of the paramedic services he applied called me for his reference, so I used the Bluetooth in my car so he could listen in. At the end of the interview, I asked if there was anything else the student had to go through to get the job as I glanced over to the passenger seat to my student with a wink. The interviewer assured me he had the job and that calling me was the last step. It brought my student to tears. This came at a time when it was difficult to get a job as a paramedic, well before the pandemic. We had seven hundred people apply for twenty spots that year.

Oddly, he said he wanted to do a shooting call before he left. Rare and critical calls such as these are better done with the safety and experience of a preceptor guiding you for your first time. I have a saying as a paramedic: "I don't want anything bad to happen, but I want to be there to patch them up if it does."

I was on the computer checking my work email when my partner said there was a multi-casualty incident going on and that we might be the next truck called. A few seconds later, the pager went off and we jumped into the ambulance.

Dispatch updated us that we were going to a shooting in a residential house with multiple patients. I turned to my student and told him he was getting his wish, and he half smiled through a look of panic. He was going to learn that these calls rev high into the redline for all first responders involved.

Police were there and hadn't cleared the house yet, so no paramedic was allowed to enter the scene. On the way, we received updates.

"First response unit cleared to access scene."

"Confirmed three patients shot multiple times."

"Two confirmed vital signs absent."

"One patient TOR."

"Two patients TOR."

"Buddy, when we get there, if there is a patient for us, we'll load them up as fast as we can and scoot!" I said to James as we flew through the streets.

As we approached the scene, we saw more cop cruisers lining the streets than I had ever seen—there must have been at least fifteen of them. We were directed into the subdivision and watched one of the ambulances leaving with a patient. Our unit was waved in to take the next patient.

We rolled our stretcher out and made haste into the house. It was total chaos. Spent shell casings everywhere, blood splattered on the floor and walls. Police, fire and paramedics scrambling to do their part. I didn't have time to process it because the last patient was ushered to me. The medic told me that there was a single gunshot wound to the head. The patient looked to be in their late twenties and was bleeding from the wound. We rushed them into the ambulance and sped off.

Our scene time was only five minutes.

After a thorough examination, we determined they had been shot once in the head. Everybody else was shot multiple times, and we could see powder and burn marks around the wound, which indicated that they were likely the shooter. The burn pattern around the entrance wound also told me that the barrel was pressed against the head before the trigger was pulled. There was no exit wound (another indicator that the gun was pressed against the head). When this happens, the bullet does not have time to develop energy if there is an obstruction against the barrel. Even a few inches is enough to give the bullet more velocity. My students and I made a great team as we got the patient intubated and established an IV before pulling into the hospital. The patient died shortly after.

The other victims were well known to the assailant. The hatred that must have gone through the patient's mind (before the bullet!) to do such a thing always amazes me. We went to the same house a year later for an unrelated call, and it was surreal to enter the house and see it fixed up. I made no mention that I was there previously.

Season: Spring
Time: 0430hrs
Weather: Nice and clear, 15°C
Area Demographic: Well-known nursing home
Dispatch Info: 85yo, unresponsive

James and I were cleaning up after a call at the hospital when dispatch asked us if we could respond to an unresponsive patient at a nearby nursing home.

My mind jumped ahead, and I thought sepsis, pre-arrest, maybe something cardiac. These were common field diagnoses that came from nursing homes. Then we got an update from dispatch:

"Uh, 2026, it's a gunshot wound to the head."

Shut the front door! James and I looked at each other with a *WTF!* So many questions ran through my head as we loaded up our stretcher and headed to the scene. *How does a gun make it into a nursing home? Was it a robbery or crime situation? Must have been smuggled in.*

We got there in three minutes, less than half the time our GPS said it would take. The police met us and said we would only have a few seconds to view the deceased as it was obvious he was dead. We went into the basement floor where the room was located, the police and they quickly opened the door.

Yep, we only needed an instant to tell the tale. There was an elderly male lying on his back. He was in only his underwear and most of his head was missing. Only his chin and one eighth circumference of his head was left. I didn't get enough time to visualize the gun or where the rest of his head was, just enough time to see that resuscitation would not be needed.

We attended a heroin overdose later that night in a bathroom at an A&W and the same officers were there. One of them said that the call came in as an unresponsive male. When the staff went to check on the individual, they found him with a gun between his legs. There was no mention if they heard a gunshot. I told my partner that if he put the gun right to his head, it would muffle the sound considerably.

Ironically, James and I watched an episode of *Forensic Files* that proved this a few nights later. They fired a .308 rifle at three feet from a pig carcass and also put it right up to the stomach. When shot against the pig, it made a decibel level equivalent to kicking a door. So, grimly, the patient's head muffled the sound of the blast. I can only imagine that the nurses heard a loud bang and went to check on him. The last thing they were suspecting was the gruesome scene they encountered.

Season: Spring
Time: 0230hrs
Weather: Cool, cloudy, 11°C
Area Demographic: Late-night café
Dispatch Info: Late twenties female, shot

We were dispatched for a non-emergent call for a woman who had been choked earlier in the night in her apartment. In this region, if the police come across a domestic where there are hands placed on someone's neck, paramedics are called to assess, potentially treat and transport the patient.

As we arrived at the scene, we saw the cops scramble to their cruisers and take off. A few seconds later, dispatch informed us that there was a shooting around the corner from us. Now we knew where the police were going.

I didn't want to leave our current patient, so my partner grabbed an extra blood pressure cuff and bandages and went up to see the patient in the apartment building while I sped to the shooting. Another crew arrived just ahead of me and was pulling the stretcher out the back. The patient was in between two doorways of the late-night café, about ten metres away. Her body was motionless, and I assumed she was VSA.

The scene was chaotic as usual. A man was yelling at the other crew that his sister had been shot. I threw a sheet underneath the patient and checked for a pulse. There was none. All of us lifted her onto the stretcher and into the back of the ambulance starting CPR. I told dispatch to alert the trauma team at the hospital. Her clothes were removed using trauma shears, and all we found was a single small gunshot wound between her third and fourth rib on the left side. It was not bleeding, was only about one centimetre long and there was no exit wound.

We dressed it with an occlusive dressing in case she had air in his lungs. After basic airway management, I used the bag valve mask to breath for the patient and then listened to breath sounds. There were none on the left side, and I suspected that a pocket of air had developed in her lung, compressing it, a condition called a tension pneumothorax. To fix it, I shoved a needle between her ribs to release the air. The hunch proved right, and I heard a rush of air exit the lung through the catheter I had put in her chest. I put a one-way valve on the catheter so that air could not re-enter, and her purple face regained colour immediately.

The trauma team met us at the ER and cracked her chest open right away. This required an incision to be made and chest spreaders to be inserted. Once in, there is a crank that spreads the chest open. It looks quite archaic. They massaged the heart outside her chest and sewed up the hole in the left ventricle. The team ran blood and even used the internal defibrillator in a last-ditch effort to start this woman's heart.

What do you know? It started beating again.

I had never seen so many stunned looks before. This happens so infrequently there was a slight pause before anything was done. For a moment they just stared at the heart. The OR was notified, and a team got ready to transport her up there, but her heart quit for the final time.

We found out later that the bullet hit the rib, made a path straight through the left ventricle and ended up in the upper abdomen. They caught it on X-ray after we left.

Gunshot calls always raise my personal tachometer. The moment they don't, I know I have become too complacent in the job and may need a readjustment of attitude. Some paramedics don't get nervous on these calls, but I'm not one of them. They keep me sharp and focused.

Chapter song selection:
"Hey Man, Nice Shot" by Filter

Chapter 11

Till Death Do Us Part

Love everlasting. Don't we all yearn for it? Finding that special someone to grow old with is one thing our society deems as the mark of true happiness. But in today's world of instant gratification and quick divorces, it seems that some long-term relationships are doomed from the get-go.

When I was first starting out in my early twenties, I overlooked the long-lasting bond between elderly couples. I could not have appreciated the luck it requires to find a compatible partner and stick out the hard times. As I matured, I began to appreciate the couples that had stayed together and were still in love. Decades pass and the love these couples share stands the test of time. Their looks have faded and their bodies are frail, but love makes them young at heart. A happiness resides in their smiles that only a lifetime of love could shape.

Season: Summer
Time: 0314hrs
Weather: Warm, clear, 16°C
Area Demographic: Seniors' apartments
Dispatch Info: 72yo male, profuse ear bleed

The patient's wife greeted us at the door with a smile and led us to her husband, who is sitting on the kitchen table holding his left ear. Apologetic for calling the ambulance at three in the morning, he explained he had been trying to stop the bleeding for over two hours. He contemplated calling a cab but didn't want to bleed all over the back seat. We told him it was no trouble, which put him at ease.

I took a gander at the wound and saw a benign abscess in his ear that probably hit a vein. We did some simple bandaging, put him on the stretcher and asked his wife if she'd like to come with us.

"I've got something important to do!" she said with a coy smile.

What could she have to do at this time in the morning? I paid it no mind, and we took the patient to the hospital. It was pretty slow, and they took him right away.

It was a beautiful early summer morning, and I was doing my paperwork on the hood of the ambulance (we did not have computers at this time, so it was actual paper!) when a cab rolled up with the patient's wife in it. She got out with a big bright bouquet of flowers. She must have gone to the twenty-four-hour grocery store around the corner. As she walked towards the emergency room entrance, she had the most beautiful smile on her face. It was filled with the anticipation of her husband receiving the gift. I was single at the time and thought to myself how wonderful it would be to be near the end of life and still have someone bring you flowers.

Season: Christmas Day
Time: 1204hrs
Weather: Cold, cloudy, -6°C
Area Demographic: Suburban residential
Dispatch Info: 76yo female, collapse, unresponsive

Working on Christmas Day is a must for paramedics. We miss out on Christmas dinner and opening presents, but most of our families understand. My family makes sure they keep a plate of dinner ready to be microwaved.

The day is usually quiet, but this Christmas Day dispatch called out for a sudden collapse. An update said that the patient was VSA. The fire department was already there, starting to run the cardiac arrest. When I got to the patient, I ran a resuscitation. The patient's heart didn't start for us, so I called for a pronouncement over the phone with a doc.

While on the phone with the doc, I took a quick look around to see if the patient and her husband had been preparing for Christmas dinner. The table was not set for a meal in the dining room, and there was no evidence of cooking in the kitchen either, so I assumed this couple was going to a family member's for Christmas dinner. My thought was, if they were having people over, I'd push to transport the patient to the hospital, that way there wouldn't be a dead body to occupy the home and force an awkward relocation of Christmas dinner.

Over a graceless conversation with the doc, we got a pronouncement. I gently covered her with a sheet and delivered the bad news to the husband who was in the kitchen.

"Sir, I'm sorry, everything that would have been done in the first few minutes in an emergency room had been done and your wife's heart hasn't started. We've stopped CPR and your wife is now dead," I said.

It's a generic canned spiel that is straight and to the point. I'm not the most empathetic at death notifications. It's one of those things I keep at an arm's reach to separate myself from the job.

But this ended up differently.

After I was finished with my universal death rambling, the man slowly reached over the kitchen table and gently held my hand, close to a bouquet of flowers. He looked at me dead in the eye and said,

"Sir, I bought these flowers three days ago for my wife. I didn't know it would be the last time I bought her flowers."

I didn't know what to say, so I didn't say anything at all. He walked over to his wife and bent over so he could gently caress her face. She still had the intubation tube from resuscitation sticking out from her mouth. I could see his mouth moving, but I could not make out any words. I didn't need to. They were the most beautiful words I couldn't hear. I called my wife, wished her a Merry Christmas and told her I loved her.

Season: Fall
Time: 1306hrs
Weather: Cool, clear, 9°C
Area Demographic: Nursing home
Dispatch Info: 90yo male, possible fractured hip

The patient's wife opened the door. She had a big smile on her face and told us her husband had fallen yesterday and had been unable to walk because of hip pain in his right side. My partner took the call and I drove. His wife asked if she could come along, and I told her it was no problem (this was a decade before COVID-19), so she seated herself next to me in the front cab. Our conversation revealed that we are from the same area of town, and she talked about how she used to serve beers to the soldiers at the armouries during the war. She fancied one in particular, and they went on a few dates, but before anything could bloom, he went off to World War II. Her mother became ill, and for many years she was her caregiver until she passed away.

Feelings of resentment and envy filled her life because she was in her mid-fifties, not married and had no children. One day, that old soldier sought her out and called her up. His wife had passed away and he was looking for new love. Wouldn't you know it? At sixty years of age, they tied the knot. She glowed with happiness from the driver's seat. The bitterness and resentment had left her.

"These past thirty years have been the best of my life," she said with a smile. "Have you ever let one get away?"

"No Ma'am, I already married her," I replied.

Make the rest of your life, the best of your life.

In a world that is disposable, automatic and full of instant gratification, it is and always will be a privilege to witness long lasting true love.

Chapter song selection:
"What a Wonderful World" by Louie Armstrong

Chapter 12

Succumbing to Mental Illness

There is a movement to change the way we view and accept mental illness. One term to interchange with suicide is "succumbing to mental illness," and if we view stage four cancer as palliative and certain end of life, then we can view suicide as someone coming to the end of their mental illness.

Suicide attempts make up a significant portion of our call volume. Most of the time, they are a call for help and not fatal. They can be aggressive, like cutting or hanging, or passive such as drug overdoses. More often than not, people just need someone to listen to them.

Whatever the chosen path to suicide is, we have to intervene. But it's not the first aid skills that help the patient, it's our compassion, empathy, communication skills and body language that save the day. Empathy and compassion are of the utmost importance, and the patient will certainly be able to call your bluff if you're fabricating it. Effective communication skills will earn the patient's trust, but poor body language, like folding your arms, will pull you in the opposite direction, aggravating the patient.

When I went to school there was no course for dealing with these calls like there are today. I learned through other paramedics' experiences and my own. When it comes down to it, paramedics need a well-rounded skill set to serve these patients effectively.

Season: Summer
Time: 0200hrs
Weather: Cool and clear
Area Demographic: Suburban house
Dispatch Info: Possible hanging

An update came across the radio as we sped to the call: there was no confirmed person hanging yet. The son of the patient received a picture text of a noose and he did not live with the patient anymore, so he called it in. With that information, I wondered if this was a bluff.

We rolled up on the scene, and the police were already there. The inner front door was open, but the outer front door was locked with a tiny deadbolt. The officer said he'd been ringing the doorbell and banging on the door. He pointed out that there were two cars in the driveway. In addition, the son said that the wife was home.

The son arrived with a key, but it was only for the inner front door, not the deadbolt on the outer front door.

Now, I know what you are thinking: break the door down. We were about to do so, but the cop pointed out that the plate glass on the outer door would not fragment like a car window, so it would be dangerous.

It looks really easy in the movies, but in reality breaking a glass door down is a huge safety hazard. You can't just smash the window and walk in. Movie glass is mostly made of sugar and water, so it explodes into small, harmless fragments. Plate glass shatters into unpredictable shards, and the edges need to be fully knocked out. Flying glass can cause injury, so safety glasses are often used. It looks bad if the first responders have to call more first responders.

There was a small, simple lock on the door that looked easy to pick. I had been practicing in my spare time, so I busted out my lock pick kit and asked permission from the cops for twenty seconds to open the lock. We were in the house in three seconds flat.

The son bolted ahead of us into the living room and I wondered to myself if the patient's bluff would be called. He entered the room first and I heard a wail of despair and agony. I anticipated that we would be walking into a grim scene. As we enter the living room, we see a man hanging from the ceiling by a noose. He was partially sitting on a small ladder with the noose tight around his neck. The rope was taught and he was barely sitting on the ladder that was underneath him. He wasn't breathing and his face was as purple as a grape.

The police officer cut the noose and the patient tumbled to the floor like a ton of bricks, smashing some glass containers in the process. Luckily, the fall was softened by the police officer partially catching him. This all happened in less than a minute in real time. A quick assessment determined he had a faint pulse, but he was not breathing. I started resuscitation with a bag valve mask, and he began to breathe on his own within a few minutes.

When he woke up, he acted as if nothing had happened. His family was crying as he sat up.

"I ain't goin' to hospital, I'm fine," he said with his arms folded in front of him like a pouting toddler.

"You don't do this to your family and get to make that decision," my partner said.

The patient reluctantly agreed, and the police informed him that he was apprehended and didn't have a choice. All the way to the hospital he gave my partner a hard time in the back of the ambulance while I drove.

No good deed goes unpunished.

Nobody said that people had to be thankful if you saved them, but this behaviour surprised me when I first started. By the end of twenty years, it had become normal.

Season: Winter
Time: 0930hrs
Weather: Cool, 10°C
Area: Urban core
Dispatch Info: Vital signs absent in car

Dispatch updated us that the caller had refused to do CPR and the patient may have been dead for a while. We didn't have much time to discuss a game plan, as the call was right around the corner. Approaching the scene, my partner and I saw a man standing beside a red car. He didn't have a sense of urgency about him as he motioned for us to come to him. He said he saw this man in the car when he went for his morning walk at about seven o'clock. When he came back two hours later, the man had not moved, and he was sure that he was dead.

A scene survey for safety revealed the patient was in the driver's seat with the seat reclined. He looked deceased because he was motionless and not breathing. His face looked like a wax figure from the 80s.

I'm gonna break the window, I thought. *Are there any hazards? It seems safe, no evidence of carbon monoxide gassing.*

The car's lights were on, but it was not running. I looked for a hose attached to the exhaust, and there wasn't one, which meant he did not use the exhaust for the suicide attempt, a common and hazardous way to commit the act.

His windows were tinted very dark and I could not see inside the car beyond the driver's seat. So for the first time in my career, I got to use my rescue knife's window breaker. The fire department showed up as I punched the window. I looked through the window to see an industrial-sized bucket in the passenger's footwell, something I could not have seen before breaking the window due to the heavy tint. Then I smelled something like a stink bomb and instantly recall a safety email I'd received.

Japanese detergent suicide!

I had kept an email about this for years to remind myself about it. The person gets common household chemicals and mixes them together, creating poison gas.

The victim is supposed to put a sign and tape the windows shut so the gas doesn't escape. This guy did neither and had blackout windows so we couldn't see. At least he locked the doors.

I conveyed this information to the firefighter and his eyes widened. He immediately notified his dispatch that we had a hazmat situation, and we evacuated the area and moved the vehicle upwind. But the damage was done and we had all been exposed to poison gas. I felt fine, but there was that sick gut feeling that I had done something wrong.

My partner and I waited in anticipation while hazmat figured out what we were dealing with. We were exposed to hydrogen sulfide, but not in toxic levels. Since the bystander had returned from his walk, the gas had dissipated to non-toxic levels. After a trip to the emergency department, my partner and I were cleared to work for the rest of the day.

I learned that immediately after mixing the chemicals, the hydrogen sulfide is at lethal levels. Two breaths at that level permanently impairs gas exchange in the lungs. You're already dead and there is nothing anybody can do. There would have been a noticeable cloud of smoke inside the car if the gas were at lethal levels. If you can smell it, it's more than likely not deadly.

When I think back to my check of the vehicle before entering, if I had seen a cloud of smoke inside the car, I wouldn't have smashed the window.

At the end of the day, my wife and I sat down and talked about the unique incident. It was only then that I thought about how dangerous the situation was, and it occurred to me that if things didn't happen the way they did, I may not be on the couch with her now. Fear gripped me and I fought back a whimper. I had to suck it up because I worked again in the morning. Who knew what the day would bring?

Season: Summer
Time: 0730hrs
Weather: Hot, clear, 30°C
Area Demographic: Apartment, urban core
Dispatch Info: Male jumper, ten stories

Jumpers are intense calls. They always land in the public view, so everybody is watching you. The pressure is tangible. Sometimes we can pronounce them right away and sometimes we can't.

We were at the hospital finishing up when the call came across the airways. I knew it was right around the corner, so I took it. I had a student medic with me for extra hands.

Upon arrival, there was already a crowd of twenty or more people around the scene and the police were taping it off. The jumper landed on the sloped entrance ramp to the underground parking at the apartment building, which created a blood trail fifteen feet long from his head. The firefighters were doing CPR, so the student and I secured his airway and applied the cardiac monitor. I knew the outcome, but we still needed to go through the motions.

We gently manipulated his head as little as possible to get an intubation tube in. Even with the slightest of manipulation, his head was like mush. After a neck collar and fracture board, we transported him to the hospital where he was pronounced shortly after.

We would find out from the police that he had been arguing with his mother when he ran off the balcony. I felt terrible for her because now she had to live with that image for the rest of her days. Although I had witnessed a gruesome death, this widow had to deal with the personal grief from the whole incident. This grief and pain wasn't mine; it was hers alone.

Keeping that in mind is how I keep my sanity. How can I feel so bad when it is someone else's loss and suffering? It's not my burden to bear.

I've responded to more than a dozen jumpers in my career. They were some of the most intense calls, but they got easier with time.

Season: Summer
Time: 0800hrs
Weather: Warm, sunny, 22°C
Area Demographic: Well-kept older neighbourhood
Dispatch Info: Elderly female, short of breath

We were driving in a beautiful part of town with older houses that people took pride in. My partner and I enjoyed looking at the homes that had a lot of character to them. Our real estate browsing was broken by the sound of dispatch calling.

I mentally prepared for a run-of-the-mill call. *We'll give some oxygen or other medications to help her breathe*, I thought. *At worst, we'll help her breathe with our bag valve mask.*

We knocked on the door, which was closed but unlocked. Nobody answered our calls of hello. Cautiously, we entered to try and find the patient. I passed through the living room while calling to see if anybody was home. Finally, we saw a slight movement coming from a rumpled-up blanket on the floor beside the couch. Unravelling the blanket yielded a young male that was unresponsive and breathing like a fish out of water.

"IT'S TIM!" my partner yells.

Tim was a fellow paramedic I had worked with more than a few times. He was an odd character, but we got along and would have great conversations when we worked together.

My partner had told me that Tim had made an attempt to take his life about two months prior. I had been off that day, so I missed the call. We kept it confidential and so did the hospital staff. Nobody knew how much Tim was hurting at the time.

What would it be like to do that call? I mentally went through it at that time to prepare myself in case it happened.

Tim was lying face down in at least two litres of blood on the floor, but we couldn't find the source of the bleeding and never did. By the time we got there, his body was in late-stage shock, which meant that his peripheral circulation had shut down. He had no veins left that I could start an IV in. I tried to keep my cool and focus on each task intently. Redirecting fear and anxiety into focus and anticipation made all difficult calls go easier. At least I fooled many people into thinking I was calmer than I really was.

My partner put the cardiac monitor on while I intubated him. His heart rate was fifty and slowing down, but by the time we got him onto the stretcher, I couldn't feel a pulse. We started CPR and hurried to the hospital.

At the hospital, we shifted Tim to the hospital bed. After a few minutes of resuscitation, the monitor still showed a flatline. I was performing CPR on my co-worker when I looked over at the ER doc for the cue to stop. I saw sympathy in his eyes. He didn't want to tell me to stop. It brought me comfort to see that the doc acknowledged how horrible this situation was. It made me feel human. He gave me the cue and I took my hands off Tim's chest. With Tim pronounced, the call was over. My management was notified and they came to the hospital.

I was taken off the road and debriefed by my management. I got the day off and went home to my girlfriend, greeting her with a sobbing cry. I had held in crying for a couple of hours, and it felt good to let it all out. Work gave my partner and me a few days off. I visited friends and family and participated in a few of my hobbies. I was fortunate to have a great support system, and within a couple of days, I felt much better.

I also learned a lot about Tim. His support system was inadequate. He had come from a broken home, with his parental figures leaving his life in his teenage years. Introverted and with few friends, paramedicine was an excellent career to break him out of his shell. During his time with us, he had met a significant other and was completing his advanced care paramedic training. Months before this incident, he had been behaving erratically at work. Arguments with hospital staff and frequent outbursts were becoming more common.

None of this information made me understand why Tim decided to end his life. Eventually, I came to understand that people who succumb to their mental illness believe that the world is better off without them. Or maybe the suffering is too much to bear on this earth. Either way, the aftershock they leave is devastating to those close to them.

I thought about this call every day for a few years. In time, I would forgive Tim for what he put my partner and me through, but it took longer to forgive myself for not being able to save him. I never treated another suicide victim the same. I had more empathy for these patients than before, so there was a silver lining in the chaos.

(Due to patient confidentiality, I never found out why we were dispatched as an elderly female, short of breath.)

Chances are that by adulthood, you know someone who has taken their own life. Take comfort that you are not alone. Help and support are out there. My best advice is to be open about it. In sharing, you'll find that others are hurting too. It will provide some comfort in the aftershock.

Chapter Song Selection:
"Jealous" by Josh Daniels

Chapter 13

The Obviously Dead

When a patient is found to have no pulse and is not breathing, the call is dispatched as VSA. As paramedics, we don't like to call these people dead. There is a mystical space between life and death where the heart and breathing have stopped but the patient hasn't passed on … yet. This is where paramedics come in to pull at this mystical void towards the side of the living.

But there are those cases where the fate of that patient has already been chosen. Patients who are so far gone that they don't need a coroner to declare death. Some of these patients have gone stiff with rigor mortis, telling us death is hours old. Or even a longer length of time has gone by and the body has been broken down by the environment, signifying decomposition.

Our work as paramedics doesn't stop there. The deceased leave behind grieving loved ones that require delicate attention. Empathy and compassion are tools that help the ones surrounding the recently departed.

Season: Summer
Time: 0800hrs
Weather: Cool, sunny, 8°C
Area Demographic: Residential house
Dispatch Info: 80yo female, vital signs absent

When paramedics get a call early in the morning for a VSA patient, it usually means they have died, unnoticed, sometime in the night. Typically, a loved one tries to wake them up unsuccessfully. With this in mind, I don't push it too hard driving to these calls.

The husband greeted us at the door and whisked us to the bedroom where the patient was.

"She was late for breakfast, so I went to wake her and she wouldn't wake up. That's when I called you guys," he said.

I got closer to the bedroom and saw her lying on her back in the bed. Her fingertips were holding the top of the covers snug below her chin, and she looked like she was comfortably sleeping.

I rushed to the patient's side and pulled off the covers to accurately assess her. The fingers that looked so snugly holding the sheets in place did not move, nor did the rest of her body. She was as stiff as a board. Rigor mortis had set in, so surely she had passed peacefully sometime during the night.

I'd like to go like that, I thought to myself.

My attention turned to the husband, who was now a widower. He told me how much he loved her.

"How long have you been married?" I asked.

"Over fifty years, sir," he answered.

"Wow, that's something to write home about," I said.

This call happened early in my career. I was in my early twenties and did not have the appreciation for a relationship that lasted that long. As the years passed, I would admire these partnerships exponentially.

Season: Summer
Time: 1200hrs
Weather: Hot, hazy, humid, 30°C
Area Demographic: Apartment, east end
Dispatch Info: Blood leaking through the floor

It doesn't take a *CSI* expert to see where this is going. Naturally, we went to the apartment that was above where the call originated. When we got there, a frantic superintendent met us in the hallway outside and told us he opened the door but did not go in because of the stench. Before I opened the door, I took a deep breath in and held it.

The only light in the apartment came from the window in which the blinds were closed. Even though it was a sunny day, I still had to use my flashlight. Yes, I could have turned the light on, but I was trying not to touch anything I did not need to because everything was a crime scene until proven otherwise. I crept into the apartment. The air conditioner in a small window unit made the place cool and comfortable. It also slowed the rate of decomposition, keeping the odour at a minimum, especially in the heat of the summer.

The patient was face down between the couch and coffee table. The feet were black, and the calves were split open from decomposition. The patient's back had exploded open and looked like green jello. I couldn't see the arms because they were tucked in beneath the chest. The head had also decomposed, melted into the floor. I could not tell for sure what race or sex the patient was, but I assumed male since the apartment belonged to a male and the outline of the body was loosely shaped like a male. Strangely, there was a transparent circumferential stain of clear fluid in the carpet three inches in diameter around him. Just beyond that, there was something peculiar: a few hundred dead flies surrounding the stain.

Those flies lived their entire life cycle around this man's body, I thought.

With no resuscitation efforts needed, we exited and talked with the superintendent.

"How the hell am I gonna clean this up?" he said, throwing his hands in the air.

"My friend has a bio cleaning business that specializes in this sort of thing. It's not cheap, but I can give you his card," I offered.

He took the card and called right away. The first thing he gave my friend was a credit card number.

Season: Spring
Time: 0200hrs
Weather: Clear, crisp, sunny, 14°C
Area Demographic: Busy urban core intersection
Dispatch Info: Self-dispatched

Somebody thought it would be a good idea to put a shelf ten centimetres above the sharps container in the back of the ambulance, which made it difficult to put discarded needles in it. So after they were installed, all units had to return to have them taken out. I was on my way to our central station to get the shelf removed when I saw traffic stopped ahead of me. There was a moving truck pulled off to the side and bystanders looking at the centre of the road. There was a motionless woman lying face down on the pavement.

I got on the radio with dispatch and told them we had a potential call on our hands. From fifty feet away, she appeared lifeless, but even at this distance, she had the most beautiful, natural, long, wavy light-brown hair. As I approached the patient, I saw a mass that was next to her purse on her torso. I thought that it might have been her intestines considering where it was located. When I got to her side, I noticed her head was crushed and cracked open. Looking at the pinkish mass again, I realized it was her brain, intact, that had somehow squeezed outside of her head. It was gruesome, but the brain looked healthy and there was little blood around her head. She looked like she was sleeping. Strangely, I imagined that if we put it back in, she would come back to life.

Dark humour is an essential paramedic survival tool.

We covered her with a blanket so that the public didn't have a view of the gruesome scene. I turned my attention to the driver who hit her, which was obvious because he was screaming in horror and looking off into space. A bystander was trying to console him, but really, what can you say? I told the bystander that he could stay and comfort him if he wanted, but it probably didn't matter.

By this time the police were on-scene and grabbed the purse that was beside ... you know. The officer held it at full arm's length and looked like he was going to throw up. We all sat in the back of the ambulance waiting for some identification to come out of the purse. I wanted to ask the officer if he found any of her thoughts in there but decided to keep that joke to myself. Things we find funny may be extremely offensive, but the general public doesn't see what we do on a regular basis. It's a coping mechanism I find necessary to balance the horrors we witness.

Later, I read in the news she was trying to make the light and was unsuccessful. The article had a picture that showed her beautiful wavy, light brown hair extended well past her waist, something I couldn't tell on scene.

Season: Summer
Time: 1600hrs
Weather: Hot, hazy and humid, 35°C
Area Demographic: Run-down apartments, east end
Dispatch Info: Patient obviously dead

Every summer, I would try to get an ice cream cone at the Stoney Creek Dairy while on duty. It was a mission since we are such a busy service. One day, my partner and I were in line contemplating what flavour we would have.

My go to, chocolate chip mint, or sweet butterscotch ripple? I pondered.

Turns out the police had come across a patient that they thought was obviously dead. Here in Ontario, paramedics are the only first responders that can declare a patient dead, so, despite having my sights on butterscotch ripple, we had to respond immediately.

This address was one of the most run-down apartment buildings in the city. It was straight out of a low-budget horror movie. The outer balconies were stained with dripping rust, there were cracks in the foundation, and it needed a paint job thirty years ago. We were the last of the first responders to show up. It looked like Christmas in summer with all the flashing lights.

As we walked up to the apartment, a man in construction gear holding his hard hat sauntered out of the apartment building entrance. He looked at all the emergency vehicles and shook his head.

"Hey man, how's it goin?" my partner shouted.

"Just another day in paradise!" he said as he headed off to work.

We laughed hysterically as we entered the elevator. The police met us outside of the apartment and apologized for calling us. They led us to the bathroom where the patient was. From the hallway, we could see that the patient was bent over the tub. His butt was facing us and the rectum was necrotic—it looked like a black button. Exposed mucous membranes decay first, so if the patient's mouth had been wide open, that would have been the first to decompose. So before we even entered the room, we knew that no resuscitation was needed.

When we got beside the patient, we saw his torso and arms inside the tub. Since decomposition had already started, our work was finished. I couldn't see any visible signs of trauma and neither could the police, so we hypothesized that he'd had a massive heart attack and collapsed into the tub, but his cause of death would never be one hundred percent certain. With no work to be done except paperwork, we left the apartment.

We hastily completed the paperwork and sped back to the Stoney Creek Dairy. This time the radio waves didn't call our truck number and we got our ice cream cones. As my partner enjoyed rocky road and I savoured my butterscotch ripple, I said, "Just another day in paradise!" We both chuckled.

Season: Early spring
Time: 1300hrs
Weather: Clear, cold, -3°C
Area Demographic: Apartment, west end
Dispatch Info: Patient vital signs absent, CPR refused

With the dispatch info, we knew we were heading into a dead body that we wouldn't be resuscitating. The landlord met us at the elevator and told us that the person in the apartment had not paid his rent since December (it was early March). Looking at me, he said we might need some Vicks VapoRub, which told me he was well-versed in decomposing bodies. When put under your nose, it nullifies the stench of a dead body. It's a great tool when entering a situation with vomit-inducing aromas.

The eviction notice was on the door of the apartment, and I noted a pile of unopened mail that had been slid underneath the door; another telltale sign that this person had been dead for a long time. We entered the apartment and noticed it was almost entirely empty. Usually, there is at least a chair or cardboard box somewhere, but there was no furniture in the living area or kitchen.

We saw the body in the hallway just outside the bathroom. Lying on his back, he was a completely preserved, mummified body. We could tell it was male, because he was naked and everything was intact. His skin was completely black from head to toe. His face was sunken in, and his mouth was wide open. You could see every rib in detail. His spine was visible through his abdomen, and the extremities were dried up and plastered to the floor. There was visible, dried-up stool in between his legs, which is common when somebody dies. There was a little blood trickling out from under his body, only about a cup and not enough to make it the cause of death. I had no idea what caused this man's death.

The strangest thing was the two open suitcases right by the door. These were the only things in this apartment. We even checked the bathroom cupboards for some supplies, but there was nothing. It looked like he was about to leave for the last time … three months ago. Nobody reported him, nobody missed him enough to call. The only reason he was found was because he owed money. It was sad and unfortunate.

We usually find photo identification somewhere around the apartment but even that was a fail. It would at least present a picture of what this person looked like before mummification. I assumed that it was in the suitcases but left that for the police. I wondered what led this person to be so secluded, but I'll never know.

After so many years, seeing dead bodies becomes normal. People ask if it bothers me, but I explain that when there is no intervention for us, it's a stress relief. These calls direct our focus and energy to loved ones if they are present or leave us to ponder what happened leading up to their death and the person they were.

Chapter song selection: "Body Count" by Ice-T

Chapter 14

The Paranormal

Paramedics are educated to be logical. We do physical assessments, and based on our findings, we treat under medical directives. The decisions we make have reasoning and logic behind them, and on rare occasions, we run into situations that require more detailed thought and experience.

Some cases have no reasoning or logic.

There are things in this world that cannot be explained. I have witnessed physical and emotional events that were so bizarre that I could not find a logical explanation for them. I didn't believe in them before they happened. Looking back with life experience, paranormal encounters don't surprise me as much. How can you be in and around death so closely and not increase your chances of having a paranormal experience?

COME RIDE WITH ME

Season: Summer
Time: 0230hrs
Weather: Warm, 14°C
Area: Urban core
Dispatch info: Elderly female, chest pain

Chest pain is one of the most frequent calls we receive, so I thought this one would be routine. We arrived on-scene and the fire department was already standing beside the patient. Standard procedure for a chest pain call is to perform a twelve-lead electrocardiogram, a detailed look at the electrical activity of the heart that can tell us if the patient is having a heart attack. It can also reveal detailed information about a person's heart conditions. In this case, the reading did not indicate that she had a heart attack.

But it was concerning.

The electrocardiogram told me that her heart was ischemic, or lacking oxygen. We do many non-urgent chest pain calls, but this one needed my full attention and skill. My focus turned to the cardiac monitor to watch for changes. As we were ready to put her on the stair chair, the patient asked me to turn off the television, so I did. I gathered her medication list, and she told me to turn off the television again. I looked, and the television was on. My first response bag was leaning against the television, so my logical mind told me it was the culprit. I pulled it away and turned the TV off for the second time.

We loaded the patient on the stair chair to extricate her from the house. For the third time, she pointed to the television and asked me to turn it off. Puzzled, I look around for the remote to see if something was pressing against it and causing this bizarre situation. The remote was sitting alone on a TV tray (something from the past you should do an internet search for if you don't know what it is!), so there is no way that something had pressed up against the button and turned the television off.

Something weird is going on!

I turned off the television again and watched it closely. One of the firefighters took the stair chair with my partner and shouted, "I'll get her to the stretcher outside." I turned my attention to my partner and the firefighter for an instant and when I looked back, the television was on again!

A cathode ray television was one that operated using a vacuum tube that projected an image on a screen. It could take time to warm up after being turned on, but when it was turned on, it made a distinct clicking sound. I realized at this time that the TV never produced the "on" sound! I shut it off again and yelled to the patient that something strange was going on with the television and I couldn't seem to turn it off. The patient took a deep breath and let out a sigh.

"That's Dan," she said. "He's a spirit that lives here, and he likes to play tricks on people."

"Okay Dan! We will take good care of her for you. I promise!" I shouted at thin air.

I was bewildered.

On the way to the hospital, the patient explained that three spirits resided in the home. Dan was a young male in his twenties who liked to cause trouble. There was a male and female couple that lived there, too, but they just appeared as apparitions, they didn't interact with the physical environment. I took extra care to do my job diligently and we made it to the hospital without incident. Dan did not follow me home and I had no further paranormal experiences from that encounter.

Season: Summer
Time: 0340hrs
Weather: Hot, 28°C
Area: Urban core
Dispatch info: 80yo female, lift assist

I mentioned the lift assist earlier as one of our most frequent calls. Many elderly people have difficulty sleeping and have to go to the washroom in the early morning hours, so it is not uncommon for us to go pick somebody off the floor.

The call was as dispatched, and we helped an elderly female who had fallen asleep in her chair and slid off onto the floor. While my partner was taking vital signs, talking to the patient and starting the paperwork, I went to look for her identification and medications.

While looking in the patient's bedroom, I noticed a bedroom at the end of the hall that was of particular interest. I peered in from the door. There was a single bed perfectly centred in the middle of the room that was meticulously made. A lavender comforter with lace trim covered it and was about three inches from the hardwood floor all around. A pillow was neatly placed on top in the centre of the headrest. The wood bed frame had no dust on it.

There was a dresser about one foot from the foot of the bed that had a thirteen-inch cathode ray television in the centre. On top of the television was a folding two-photograph picture frame with an elderly man in each of the photos. I assumed this to be her husband. On top of the photo was a pristine fedora hat without a speck of dust on it. There was a window facing the street with satin blinds that were neatly separated on each side with bows. On the opposite wall was a bookshelf that housed books all of the same size. I had an uneasy feeling of not wanting to be in the room as I entered, and that feeling quickly changed to "You don't belong here!" so I left.

My partner was obtaining the patient's signature for a refusal to transport to the hospital, and I asked, "Is that your husband's room? It's the cleanest, tidiest room in the house."

"Yes, he passed away five years ago. He certainly liked everything clean, it was hard to keep up. I keep that room in memory of him, and I keep it tidy," she replied.

We asked her if there was anything we could do, and she replied that we could pick up the newspaper from the floor. I neatly re-folded and placed it on the armrest of her chair. She sat in her chair facing the living room television and quickly fell asleep, snoring almost instantly.

I walked into the deceased husband's bedroom and placed myself at the opposite corner of the room facing the door. I talked my partner into coming into the room and within a few seconds, a look of uneasiness came across his face. I scurried across the room and grabbed his wrist as he tried to leave. I mischievously looked him in the eye and asked him to stay a little longer, but that feeling of not belonging there overcame us both and we darted for the ambulance.

"Dude, the look on your face when you entered the room was priceless! You stopped in your tracks, stunned," I said.

"I wanted to get out of there ASAP, but you were holding my wrist!" James said, only slightly angry.

I looked at the window of the apartment that was facing the roadway and saw a faint dark shadow move across the window. The blinds with the bows swayed! I put the ambulance in drive and sped off quickly.

Season: Summer
Time: 0300hrs
Weather: Warm, no wind, 15°C
Area Demographic: Upscale suburban home
Dispatch Info: Intruder, person in the home with increased confusion

As the info came across the airwaves, my partner and I gave each other a confused look. With no medical emergency, we wondered why we were dispatched. The only additional information we were provided with was to wait for police before entering.

When we arrived on the scene, the firefighters were already leaving the house. They told us that the police didn't even respond there anymore because the old woman was crazy and they had never found an intruder. The firefighters also told us that they were tired of coming there countless times.

We entered the house, and an elderly lady greeted us. After talking to her for a few minutes, we realized she had dementia. She mentioned that a man was in the room lying on the couch and that he was still in the house somewhere. She wanted us to go look for him.

We decided to assess her first and make sure she checked out medically. Other than being a little confused, her vitals were good and we couldn't find anything out of the ordinary with the cardiac monitor. After talking with her, we discovered she was a widow. Strangely, her confusion disappeared when she talked about her husband or anything to do with the past. She asked us again to look through the house just to make sure it's vacant. Since it was three in the morning and the radio was relatively quiet, we entertained her request. I let dispatch know what we were up to and told the patient that we may have to leave if another call comes in.

We started in the basement.

"Stevie, I don't like this," my partner said. "The hairs on the back of my neck are standing up!"

"I'm not feeling anything yet, let's keep looking," I replied.

The basement stored a few old dressers and a piano. There was also a bunch of junk like all basements have. But there was something that I'd never seen before in a basement—a wall that had a few bricks missing that led into another room. We peered into the room and saw some outdated furniture—that was all.

Pretty anticlimactic.

While clearing the first floor, I noticed something peculiar. Every ten feet there was a melee weapon of some type—sewing scissors, a butter knife, staplers—on tabletops. Canes and umbrellas were leaning against the walls. Whether a person was in the house or not, this woman was ready for a fight to defend herself. It made me diligent in my search because, no matter what I believed, this woman believed that someone was in her home. For me to leave without the patient's needs met was a non-starter; I needed to do a thorough check to make sure there was no one to harm her.

We checked closets and underneath the beds, but there was no intruder to be found. As I entered the final room, the temperature dropped significantly. So much so, that I could see my breath.

It's summertime, I shouldn't be able to see my breath! There's no furniture or objects in this room, strange.

There was a small walk-in closet, the last place to check in the entire house. Now the hairs on the back of my neck were standing up, and the feeling of uneasiness my partner felt in the basement came over me. I entered the closet and felt a slight wind. There were no vents in the closet so I was confused about where it was coming from. There was a small trapdoor at the end of the closet, and man did I want to open it! That's when I felt something that did not communicate with words but with emotion.

Don't come near this door.

It was pure terror.

I'm gonna open that door!

As I approached the trapdoor, the wind got stronger along with that feeling of terror. The wind got so forceful that I couldn't keep my eyes open anymore. Okay, I got the message.

I backed out of the closet and stepped out into the hallway to catch my breath. The feeling of terror and the wind were instantly gone. My partner and I reconvened on the first floor and told the woman that we couldn't find anyone. She thanked us and we left, but I wasn't sure we were leaving her alone...

The aforementioned account is documented in season 1, episode 8 of *Paranormal 911* if you care to indulge.

These experiences are more common than you would think. In fact, when I shared them with other medics, they told me of their own paranormal experiences. If you don't have an encounter, then you get to not believe. Believe me ... I'd rather not believe.

Chapter song selection:
"Ghostbusters" by Ray Parker Jr.

Chapter 15

That's Not in My Job Description!

When I signed up for the paramedic program at Fanshawe College in 1999, I had no idea what I was getting myself into. I thought being a paramedic was simple: drive an ambulance with lights and sirens, take care of patients with medical emergencies, then drive to the hospital.

It's not always that simple.

I couldn't possibly know the number of diverse encounters I would have as a paramedic…

Season: Spring
Time: 1900hrs
Weather: Mild, 15°C
Area Demographic: Wealthy neighbourhood with lots of elderly people
Dispatch Info: Unconscious diabetic

I had completed treatment on an unconscious diabetic. Usually these patients have low blood sugar, so we give them sugar through the veins and they wake up. This call went like clockwork and within a few minutes the patient was awake and talking. The next part in treatment is to stand by and watch them eat a complex carbohydrate to make sure they don't drop their blood sugar later on.

The parents of the patient that owned the house told me not to leave the door open because their dog could escape. Now, this dog was a spunky two-year-old purebred Doberman named Buddy—not a dog that an eighty-year-old couple should not be taking care of. Buddy was friendly and boisterous, and they, unsuccessfully, tried to keep him upstairs. When I opened the door to put back one of my response bags, Buddy made a run for it. Out into the streets he went. I felt guilty because there was no way that the elderly couple was going to get this dog back without some help.

So out into the streets I went.

One of the other medics, Josh, joined the chase and brought a ball. We tried all the tricks we could think of—throwing the ball, pretending to have a treat in hand, even chasing him for fun. At no time did I feel the dog was going to harm me. He would charge us, then at the last split second, dart off to the side and take off.

After about twenty minutes, I could see he was getting tired, so I ran flat out as fast as I could. The dog let me think I was gaining on him before I gassed out. I was quickly panting and out of breath, hands on my knees. I was also having more fun than I would like to admit.

That's when things took a turn.

Buddy fled out onto a sixty kilometre an hour rural highway. He was like a kid in a candy store chasing the cars, except they were either coming to a screeching halt or swerving out of the way. Surprisingly, one guy stopped and chatted with us, offering to take Buddy home. The dog was on its hind legs, head and front feet in the window.

This is my chance!

I tried to sneak up on him, but he heard me and darted off.

Buddy decided to stop and eat some grass. We were by the side of the road on an embankment with a drainage system. Once again, I approached cautiously but from the front this time. Josh approached from the back, but I waved him off. I had an idea. I don't know where this came from, but it seemed logical at the time. I got on all fours and pretended to eat grass just like he was. I acted like I was his best friend. Slowly, I moved sideways (still on all fours) towards him. Buddy lifted his head to look at me. For some reason, I made chewing motions and an "Mmm" sound. He seemed to have a *duh okay* look on his face and continued eating grass. I moved even closer, continuing to pretend to eat grass. Now I was an arm's length away. I can't imagine how ridiculous this must have looked from the side of the road: a paramedic on all fours pretending to eat grass beside a rambunctious Doberman. Later, Josh told me he should have filmed it.

It was time to make my move. Being a martial artist for over thirty years, I knew how to take down humans safely, but I had never attempted to apprehend a dog. Most importantly, I did not want to hurt Buddy…

I lunged with my left hand over his body while simultaneously grasping his collar with my right hand. I pulled him towards me and cradled him close as we slid and rolled down the embankment. The region had a copious amount of rainfall and the storm drain was full. Buddy and I plunged into the stagnant, muddy drain water and I let go of Buddy's torso and kept hold of his collar.

If Buddy could speak, he would have said, "That was fun! Can we do it again?"

His owner had now found us on the side of the road. He put Buddy in the back seat of his truck while scolding him. Back at the house, the elderly couple thanked me and let me clean the sewage and mud off of my arms. Since I was covered in mud and smelled like sewage, I put myself out of service. At the station, I showered and changed, ready for the next one.

Season: Winter
Time: 0015hrs
Weather: Cold, 1°C
Area Demographic: Urban east
Dispatch Info: Male, intoxicated

The caller emerged from a crowd of smokers and waived us down. We saw a man lying face down on the grass beside the sidewalk.

"Hey guys, this is they guy, I tried to wake him up but couldn't," the caller said.

"Thanks for doing that, most people never approach the patient. By the way, what is going on here?" I asked, pointing to the crowd.

"Stag and doe!" he said.

"He's not a part of it, is he? Nobody knows him?" I asked.

"Nah!" he said, returning to the party.

The patient looked pretty rough. A beat-up old leather jacket and dirty work jeans made his wardrobe whereas most of the people that were smoking outside were dressed well and clean.

We approached the patient, and I couldn't tell if he was breathing. Even five feet away in the open air, I could smell the booze on him. I bent down, gently shook him and yelled to wake him up. After he arose, my partner asked him if he was okay. He admitted he'd had a few too many, and we helped him to his feet. I asked permission to take his vital signs, and he politely agreed, so I went to grab the cardiac monitor from the ambulance.

Now I don't know what happened in the ten seconds it took me to do this, but Mr. Hyde indeed showed up. When I approached him this time, he used a popular four-letter word and told me where to go. I complied and backed away. I asked him if he would sign a form refusing treatment, and I got the same four-letter word. My partner and I looked at each other and shrugged. We prepared to leave and notify the police.

"I'm gonna show you what it is like to run out into traffic," he mumbled.

I didn't take him seriously, but he slowly stumbled out into traffic. A car swerved, barely missing him. I ran onto the road and pulled him back onto the sidewalk. Firmly but still politely, I pleaded with him not to do that again. The outside smokers from the stag and doe are entirely into it now.

"Let em go! We wanna see him get hit!" one yelled.

Early in my career there were no cell phones that could record video, so it was easier to say what was on my mind. This call happened in the digital age, so I assumed I was being filmed at all times. As such, we did not reply to the crowd—it's just safer that way. Suddenly, the patient said he just wanted to go home. He pointed down the street and started walking that way.

I followed him for a few steps, knowing that a car was approaching on the curb lane, and I watched his body language. He was preparing to leap out in front of it. As the car got nearer, he stepped closer to the edge of the street. I crept behind him and as he tried to leap and grab his thick leather jacket from behind.

"Stop!" I yelled.

He tried to take my head off with a big right hand, and I was almost caught off guard, but my martial arts kicked in and I blocked his punch. He instantly followed up with a left, but I got inside both of his arms and grabbed a hold of his jacket again.

My partner and I always referenced a quote from the movie *Road House*: "Be nice, until it's time not to be nice." This was one of those times. My partner called a 10-2000—a Mayday call to get the police to come to our location because we were in grave danger.

I stepped to his left, foot swept him to the ground and got a high mount on him. I held his arms down as he tried to pepper me with punches from the bottom. This man was in his early forties, 6'2" and over two hundred pounds. It was real work keeping him on the ground

"BEAT THE SNOT OUT OF HIM!" an onlooker shouted.

"I'm not trying to hurt you, I'm doing this for your own safety," I said to the man.

At no time did I decide to strike or injure the man.

After what seemed like forever, the police rolled up. The cruiser stopped about thirty metres away and shone a light on us. When the officer realized what was going on, I heard the engine roar and tires squeal. The officer parked as close to us as possible and promptly jumped out of the cruiser.

I told him what happened, and he said, "Good job, we'll take it from here."

If I thought this drunk guy was being rude to me, it was nothing compared to how he treated the cops. He started off by calling them pigs and then insulted them about how they hide behind their badges. It went downhill from there. These cops didn't let him get to them, and into the back of the cruiser he went.

The smoker crowd had thinned out as we went back to the ambulance.

"Why didn't you let the guy get smoked by a car? That would have been awesome to see!" one of the onlookers asked me.

"What wouldn't be awesome is the car veering and taking all of you out," I replied.

"Oh, I didn't think of that. Thanks," he said.

"No problem," I said.

Back at base, the excitement wore off and I was exhausted. I got the call detail times from dispatch and found out it was only three minutes from the time the 10-2000 transmission was made to the police arriving. Bruce Lee said that it was too long, and he was right.

Why am I so exhausted and emotionally shocked? I wondered to myself.

I had fought competitively for fifteen years and had never felt drained like this. There were a few factors. We did not get the time or proper information to mentally prepare for the actions of the patient. If the call were dispatched as an aggressive patient, we would have been more ready for it. But in this case, dispatch didn't know the patient would become violent, nor did I. Also, we were alone. I'd been attacked before, but the patients were much smaller, or police and fire were there.

But the main factor was that I was actually in danger. There were no referees to stop the fight. Nonetheless, I was relieved with the outcome and glad nobody got hurt.

Season: Summer
Time: 0230hrs
Weather: Warm, 23°C
Area Demographic: Urban core
Dispatch Info: Female overdose, unresponsive

We were deep into the wave of the opioid crisis when call after call was respiratory arrest and Narcan, a narcotic used to reverse or reduce the effects of various opioids. Not only was heroin present in the drugs, but other synthetics that were more potent. Popcorn, purple heroin and carfentanyl were just a few of the drugs floating around.

We were called to an unresponsive female overdose. Police were on-scene and gave us an update.

"Hey Stevie K, this one just got released from prison a few days ago and has been on a bender," Officer Bill, whom I knew well, said; he always used my nickname. "She's got a violent criminal history, so I'd be careful waking her up."

I could tell from a few feet away that the patient was not breathing. When we got to her side, I confirmed she was in complete respiratory arrest. Bill handed me a bottle of OxyContin (a common opioid), the culprit for the night. Due to her violent history, I did not give the drug Naloxone. She could wake up fighting and then we would have another problem on our hands. Instead, I intubated her and let the hospital take it from there.

After cleaning up and doing some paperwork, one of the nurses informed me that I'd missed something in my advanced assessment. The staff knew I had recently passed my advanced care paramedic certification and there was a coy smirk on his face. Perplexed, I entered the resuscitation room to see what I might have overlooked. Another nurse, smiling, presented me with a little cat figurine that I recognized to be a Maneki-neko, a cat with a waving hand that symbolizes good fortune—you've seen them in Asian restaurants for sure! The cat was hollow and had a little baggy attached to it which looked like it housed crack cocaine.

"How did I miss this, guys?" I asked, perplexed.

"When we gave her the urinary catheter, we found it waving from her vagina. You didn't notice the pussy in the pussy, Stevie K?" he said, bursting out laughing.

"That's not in my job description!" I replied with a laugh.

A paramedic's job is more diverse than I could have ever imagined. These anomalies keep the job interesting. In the back of my mind, I always remember that anything could happen at any time. It's not fear, it's awareness. The more aware I am, the better prepared I can be for any situation.

Chapter song selection:
"Working for the Weekend" by Loverboy

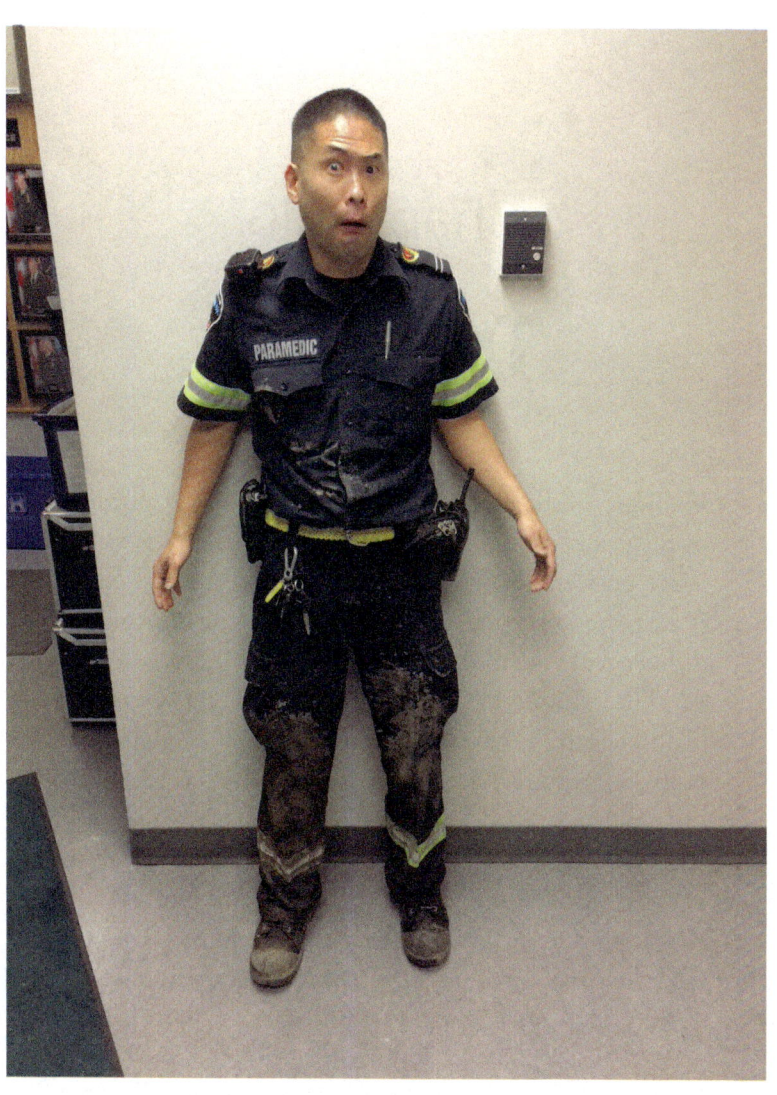

Covered in sewage from the drainage ditch after wrestling with Buddy. I smelled awful.

Chapter 16

Trauma

I still get a little excited when I hear a trauma call come over the airwaves. They are high energy and fast paced. Time on-scene matters. In critical cases, the end result is surgery, so staying on the scene too long can be the difference between life or limb.

The critical thinking and decision-making process is different from medical calls. You have to find and fix problems as you go, sometimes not moving forward until the problem is fixed.

In a medical call, you might administer medication and see where things go from there. On a trauma call, you might have to stabilize a fracture before moving on while keeping in mind that you have to get to the hospital quickly. Here are a few cases that stuck out in my mind.

Season: Early spring
Time: 1830hrs
Weather: Cool, cloudy, 10°C
Area Demographic: Urban core railway
Dispatch Info: 9yo struck by a train

I knew my relief would be waiting for me at the base by the time we got back. We had just offloaded our patient at the hospital that put us into overtime. Then the radio crackled with something significant.

"9yo struck by train, severe leg injury with severe bleeding."

I could have ignored the radio and went home, but there are calls we drop everything and rush to. Kids sustaining significant trauma is one of them. I always told myself that if there was a child in need, I would do everything I could to help. I carried that throughout my career.

I knew that with my partner driving we could make it there in five minutes. I shot him a look, and without saying anything we bolted for the ambulance. We received updates from dispatch en route.

"Leg bleeding severe, possible amputation."

Tourniquet may have to be applied, I thought. *Must be bad, kid will be scared, might need fluid and morphine. How am I going to put this nine-year-old at ease?*

As we pulled up, we saw the patient with a couple of police officers down by the train tracks about 250 metres from the roadway. I was impressed by the fast police response. They are always first when there is a kid involved. That's the way it is in Hamilton.

We got to the train tracks and James got a crazy idea.

"Dude, I'm gonna mount the tracks," he said.

"Are you crazy? Can we clear it? And what if a train comes?" I said frantically.

"Police will have it shut down, and I know we can clear it 'cause the CN service trucks do!" he said confidently.

Bouncing up and down on the train tracks, we made our way up to the scene. As we approached, I saw one of my favourite police officers. I call him Karl Urban because he looked so much like the actor. As I exited the ambulance, I heard the little boy screaming in horror and pain. He looked at me and screamed out for me to help him. Multitasking is essential for a call to run efficiently, so I assessed his leg and asked what happened at the same time. He explained that he was playing by the train and tried to get away but tripped. This translated to either train jumping or playing chicken with a train. There was no time for judgement.

Although his leg injury was evident (a picture I'll never forget), it was important to make sure that I didn't miss another serious injury. I completed a quick head to toe and, luckily, he only had that one isolated injury. Karl Urban had already applied a combat tourniquet to the patient's leg, saving his life.

The injury was a jumbled mess. What I could identify was that the tibia and fibula were sticking out about six inches and that the foot was twisted around 270 degrees. Much adipose and internal tissues were exposed about five centimetres below the knee. It was almost completely ripped off.

I took some dressings and bandages and bundled everything together. I tried to make a splint for it, but it was faster to splint the leg with three sets of hands. I remembered all first responders were on deck as we got the patient to the stretcher. I had a student with me that had exemplary communication skills, so I let her console the patient while I did all the technical work.

"So what are you doing in school right now?" the student asked.

"Science, I hate it!" the patient replied.

"I used to, but now I love it," the student countered.

The dialogue put the patient at ease and distracted him from the situation. That gave me the opportunity to get some pain relief on the way.

The pediatric trauma team as well as the vascular and orthopedic surgery were waiting for us. The vascular surgeon confirmed that the femoral artery was severed, which meant he would have bled out in minutes.

When I got the dispatch times for the call, I discovered it took us six minutes to get there. The police officer who got there first and applied that tourniquet saved his life, so I called his staff sergeant to let him know what a great job his officer did. He ended up getting an article on the CBC for his excellent work.

Season: Fall
Time: 1730hrs
Weather: Clear, cool, 12°C
Area Demographic: Work site at a parking lot
Dispatch Info: Man impaled on a pole

I was at the hospital when I heard "impaled" on the radio and my ears perked up. The call was located on the scene of a construction site. Since impalement calls are extremely rare, I offered to help out and sped off to the scene.

Another ambulance crew, the fire department and police were already. I saw a solidly-built middle-aged man on all fours on the ground just outside a construction trailer.

The crew on-scene said the patient was exiting the trailer when he slipped on the stairs. Falling backward, he hit the back of his thigh on a three-foot-high support pole for the staircase. It went in through the back of his mid-thigh and came out at the top of his buttocks.

So here was this solid middle-aged man on all fours with a pole stuck out of his butt. What a strange sight. Something I never thought I would see.

I began by building rapport.

"Sir! I'm Steve. I'm going to tell you everything we are going to do before we do it, okay?" I said.

The fire department disconnected the support pole from the stairs with a hacksaw. The pole weighed a few pounds, but I decided that the only way to stabilize it was to hold it in place with a few sets of hands. In school, they teach you cribbing and splinting techniques. But like most calls, this case wasn't in the textbook, so I had to think on my feet.

I took an additional medic to the hospital for an extra set of hands. I couldn't give him morphine due to his low blood pressure, but we still had to assess his pain, which required asking what the pain feels like. There are common descriptive words including "stabbing," "burning," "dull," "achy," "tearing," etc.

"What does it feel like?" the other medic asked.

"Feels like I got somethin' stuck up my ass!" he replied angrily.

I had to turn away and laugh while holding the pole in place.

After we handed the patient over, a doc who I knew well peered in.

"What's going on here?" she asked.

"Have a look for yourself doc," I said. "Just another pain in the ass."

Season: Fall
Time: 1100hrs
Weather: Cool, 11°C
Area Demographic: Steel making facility
Dispatch Info: Arm injury

Dispatch didn't give us much detail on the radio other than the steel plant's medical facility said that the arm was severely injured and that it was purple. That sparked interest. My partner and I always talked about a field diagnosis on the way to significant calls. We knew that almost anything could have injured him, but what it turned out to be was the furthest thing from our minds.

As we arrived at the scene, a security vehicle with emergency lights flashing guided us to the medical building. As we wheeled the stretcher into the medical room, there was a man who looked to be in his forties sitting on the exam table. His right arm was three times the size of his left and was purple. I'd never seen anything like it before, and as we loaded him onto the stretcher, I gathered the story about how this happened.

"We have a vacuum that picks up the slag from the steel process," his co-worker said.

"K, I know what slag is, the metal impurities from making steel. It's heavy, right? And that would mean the vacuum is super powerful, right?"

The co-worker nodded.

Damn, this is super serious.

"I wasn't paying attention and my arm got caught in the vacuum," the patient said.

"How long was it in the vacuum for?" I asked.

"About forty-five seconds, not a minute," he answered.

It was long enough to cause severe damage to his arm. He had no palpable pulses or feeling in his arm. It was the first time I'd ever seen what we call compartment syndrome in an arm. It more commonly happens in the legs. When I patched to the trauma centre, they said they had never heard of that in an arm, and the tone of voice was doubtful.

Upon arrival, we offloaded him to a trauma bay. The triage nurse told me that ortho didn't believe our story.

After getting coffee, we peered back into the bay. They were preparing him for an emergency escharotomy to treat compartment syndrome. Chalk one up for the medics.

Season: Summer
Time: 1600hrs
Weather: Warm, 20°C
Area Demographic: Highway exit
Dispatch Info: Pedestrian struck

It was my first day on the job, and I remember this one like it was yesterday even though it has been over twenty years. It was a bright, warm summer day. I was at base washing dishes when the pager went off for the call. It was my turn to attend, so I was in the passenger seat.

The location was right around the corner, and we could see the body was already covered in a tarp with a pair of legs sticking out from underneath. There was a six-tonne truck near the scene, which I assumed had struck the victim, as well as an overturned bicycle. I got out and saw a piece of hair and skull about a square centimetre on the ground. My partner said that an eyeball was staring him in the face.

We approached the scene and saw grey matter leaking out from the tarp. This meant there was an open spinal or cranial wound and the fluid was leaking out. It also indicated the patient was dead. A man whom I assume was the driver was leaning against the six-tonne trunk and sobbing. A teenage boy was also crying near the tarp. In real time, this was only about a minute.

"How do you do this every day?" a bystander asked me.

"Ma'am, this is my first day, so I don't really know," I said.

The police said that the boy was on his bicycle and fell directly under the path of the truck where his head was run over. The teenage boy was his friend and witnessed the whole thing. My partner said we would transport the patient's friend to the hospital and victim services would meet us there.

I was up to attend, so I sat in the back. All the boy did was cry, and I didn't know what to say. So I said nothing for a while. Eventually, I just started to talk about what would happen when we got to the hospital. I put my hand on his shoulder as it was all I could think of to do with my one day of experience.

We arrived at the hospital, and I handed him off to victim services. A couple of medics asked me if I was okay, and I said I was. The one good thing that came out of this was that I knew that I could take a gruesome call and keep on going.

Later that year, we would pass the spot where that teenage boy lost his life. A wreath had been placed there in his memory. I returned to that spot ten years later to place a single rose on the memorial in remembrance of that day. At that moment, I thought of all that had happened in my journey as a paramedic and all I would have to face until retirement. I recalled the positive of knowing I could handle a traumatic call on the first day of my job and the circumstances that happened for me to see that. I carry that with me to this day.

Chapter song selection:
"Accidents" by Alexisonfire

Chapter 17

Lucky

You can't count on luck, but luck counts. Many people rely on it with complete ignorance—just look around. How many people are distracted driving? Do you know someone who drinks and drives? Or that friend who still refuses to wear their seat belt? Of course, nothing tragic happens to these people.

Until it does.

I don't know the statistics, but the chances of getting into a motor vehicle collision where you need your seat belt is slim. Personally, I haven't been in a collision where my seat belt was needed. They were all pretty minor, yet I always wear it. It was only luck that kept me safe. But I believe you can increase your luck by increasing your chances. Increasing your chances means taking precautions like not drinking and driving, and wearing your seat belt. Despite not taking safety measures, these next few patients survived. In each case I had to reason why they weren't severely injured or dead.

Season: Summer COVID-19
Time: 0300hrs
Weather: Mild, calm, warm, 20°C
Area Demographic: Niagara Escarpment
Dispatch Info: Single car collision at Law and Tote

We got info that bystanders heard a loud car crash at the intersection of Law and Tote. As we came to that intersection, there was no car to be seen but we could hear the faint cries of a female. Law street was parallel to the base of the escarpment, which is about ninety metres tall on average. It has a steep drop at the top followed by a gradual slope at the bottom. The screams were coming from about halfway up the escarpment. My partner and I couldn't tell how far up because it was too dark and that part was not lit at night.

Dispatch updated us that there was evidence at the top of the escarpment that the car had driven off the ledge! We were given a new location at the top of the escarpment and got back into the ambulance and headed up. Upon arrival we saw that the fence had been broken through.

I had just bought a new thousand lumens flashlight with a good throw distance and I put it to use. When I shone it through the broken fence I could clearly see the car had blown through the fence and taken off the tops of two trees in succession.

The cries of the woman were louder now. It looked safe to start walking down the escarpment, so I did. This was near the beginning of the pandemic, so I had my North 7700 respirator on. This was a pretty physical call, and I was panting within a few minutes. In addition, I had a helmet and safety vest on. It was like moving through a jungle to get to the patient.

I came to a spot where there was a sudden steep drop to the part of the escarpment that became more level. The car and the woman were only about thirty metres from the base of the slope. I reached for a tree root to brace myself while I got my footing on the ledge, but it was slippery. I lost my grip and footing and slid down five metres or so, cutting my forearm in the process. It wasn't serious, not even a stitch would be needed, but it was full of dirt and would need attention later.

I was probably supposed to wait for the fire department to figure out what to do, but that would have taken too long and this was much more fun. I approached the car and the victim, but was unable to tell the extent of the damage to the car because it was so dark. Even with a bright flashlight, I couldn't see the entire car. The patient had gotten themselves out of the vehicle and was walking around looking for help.

She had a nice dress on, her hair was done and she was wearing make-up (which was now smeared all over). She smelled of perfume and alcohol. I did a thorough assessment and concluded that she only had a moderate head laceration that would require a few stitches. This person did not break a single bone in her body. As far as I could tell, she was going to be just fine. As we brought the patient out to the waiting ambulance, the news crews were waiting to film us. We rolled emergency lights and sirens to the trauma hospital anyway due to the mechanism.

Upon arrival at the hospital, the trauma team was waiting for me. I could tell by the look on their faces that they had a hard time believing the story. I couldn't blame them. How do you fly off the top of an escarpment that is ninety metres tall, take off the tops of trees and survive? Well, I thought about it and came to the conclusion that the trees slowed and braced her descent. The car came off a section of the escarpment that had a slope that started high up, so the drop wasn't that much. The car hit the front first and rolled (I saw the damage on the evening news).

Despite what I stated in the introduction to this chapter, this woman was wearing her seat belt. Had to have been, otherwise there would have been much more collateral damage.

Season: Summer
Time: 0800hrs
Weather: Clear, cool
Area Demographic: 100km/h highway
Dispatch Info: Single vehicle in the ditch with one ejected, possible pediatrics involved

Sunday morning can be quiet for the ambulance usually until about 11 a.m. Prior to that time, I call it Saturday night clean up. The leftover drug overdoses and drunks get found lying around the streets and we pick them up. I assumed that this encounter would be someone who was still drunk from the night before. I assumed wrong.

There were conflicting reports on the location of this collision. Not only where it was but on what side of the highway. This is the case many times when responding to the highway. Typically, a bystander calls it in and gives a rough area where the collision might be. I'm not blaming them for not being able to pinpoint a position where the accident occurred—most people don't know their exact location at a given time while driving.

In these cases, I like to enter the highway one exit behind the location, if possible. That way there is higher chance of locating the accident. I looked on my side of the highway and my partner looked on the other side. Eventually, we saw that it was on the other side of the highway coming the opposite way. The damage was severe. The roof of the car had been partially torn off, and the hood was smashed up against the windshield. The fire department was on-scene but no paramedic yet.

I stopped and let my partner out. Safely and with much caution, he crossed the highway. Luckily, it wasn't that busy early on Sunday morning. I passed the collision and used those turnarounds that have signs that say, "Authorized vehicles only." Jumping out of the ambulance, I saw that all the occupants of the car were, miraculously, walking around. My partner had determined that one of the occupants wasn't wearing his seat belt, so we decided to take that patient. I took a quick pic of the wreck without examining it and would analyze it later during a spare moment on the trip to the hospital. The patient walked up to me casually.

"Hey man, can you tell me what happened?" I asked.

"Uh, I flew out of the car and rolled halfway up the embankment," the young man said.

"Were you wearing your seat belt?" I asked.

"Uh, no" he said.

"Did you hit your head or lose consciousness?" I asked.

"No, I just rolled up the embankment pretty hard," he replied.

Bewildered that he was not more seriously injured, I put a cervical collar on him and put him on the stretcher.

In the ambulance, I noted that he had dried grass and minor abrasions all over his body and his clothes were tattered and torn. But I could not find a broken bone or a single laceration that would require stiches.

Off to the hospital we went.

Considering the high speed and damage to the car (part of the mechanism of injury), we activated lights and sirens and made haste to the emergency room. When we got there, I talked to the triage nurse behind the window. We do this when we want to say things that we don't want the patient to hear. I showed the triage nurse the picture and explained the situation. She could not believe the extent of the injuries either. The nurse scolded the patient by telling him she has a son his age and he should have been wearing his seat belt. The trauma team gave him a once over and I left for the next call.

On the next shift, I popped in to get an update. There was no alcohol involved. These boys were on a feeder team for professional football and were heading to practice. The nurse said they were very thankful and left with a new sense of life. I hope to see them in the NFL or CFL someday.

Season: Summer
Time: 2300hrs
Weather: Clear, warm, 23°C
Area Demographic: 100km/h highway
Dispatch Info: Single car in the ditch, rollover, patient trapped.

We were far away from this call and it took a few minutes to get there. Upon arrival, we saw a single vehicle rolled over on its passenger side. There were bystanders with flashlights who seemed to be keeping the car from tipping over by holding the roof. I approached and they shouted that there was someone in the car who was alive.

I looked in the car to see a man on the front passenger side by the window. His head was outside the front passenger window and pinned between the ground and the door.

"Can you wriggle your head out?" I asked the patient.

"No!" the patient replied in a muffled tone.

"K guys, let's push the car and relieve the pressure on his head," I said to two of the bystanders.

"Does that feel better?" I asked the patient.

I get back a muffled, "Yeah!"

The fire department arrived at the scene and I gave them an update. When safety permits, we try to get inside and start treatment, but in this case it was clear that entry to the vehicle was too dangerous. The firefighters asked me to step back so they could extricate the patient before we treated him. I always loved watching them do this. This crew communicated well and stayed task-focused.

They started by putting airbags and cribbing underneath for stabilization. Then the jaws of life came out along with a windshield saw. In a few minutes, the patient was on a backboard, cervical collar on and handed over to us.

Upon examination we determined that there were some significant lacerations to his head that would need stitches, but no obvious fractures. He told us that he remembered everything and didn't lose consciousness. He swore there was no alcohol involved and that he was wearing his seat belt. I didn't believe he could have ended up where he was if he was wearing his seat belt. Many people deny the obvious thinking they won't get in trouble.

We sped off to the hospital and called a trauma alert. Later, we found out that he was just fine after receiving his stitches. My partner and I pondered this for a while over coffee. Our conclusion was that because it had been raining, the ground was still soft so it cushioned the crash and didn't squish his head like a grape. Perhaps if it were a dry spell, the outcome would have been different. The rain was lucky, but I'd rather rely on my seat belt.

Rather than take chances, I'd like to increase chances of survival. This means being safe when I can and taking precautions both inside and outside of the world of paramedicine. The real challenge will be passing this on to my kids.

Chapter song selection: "Get Lucky" by Daft Punk

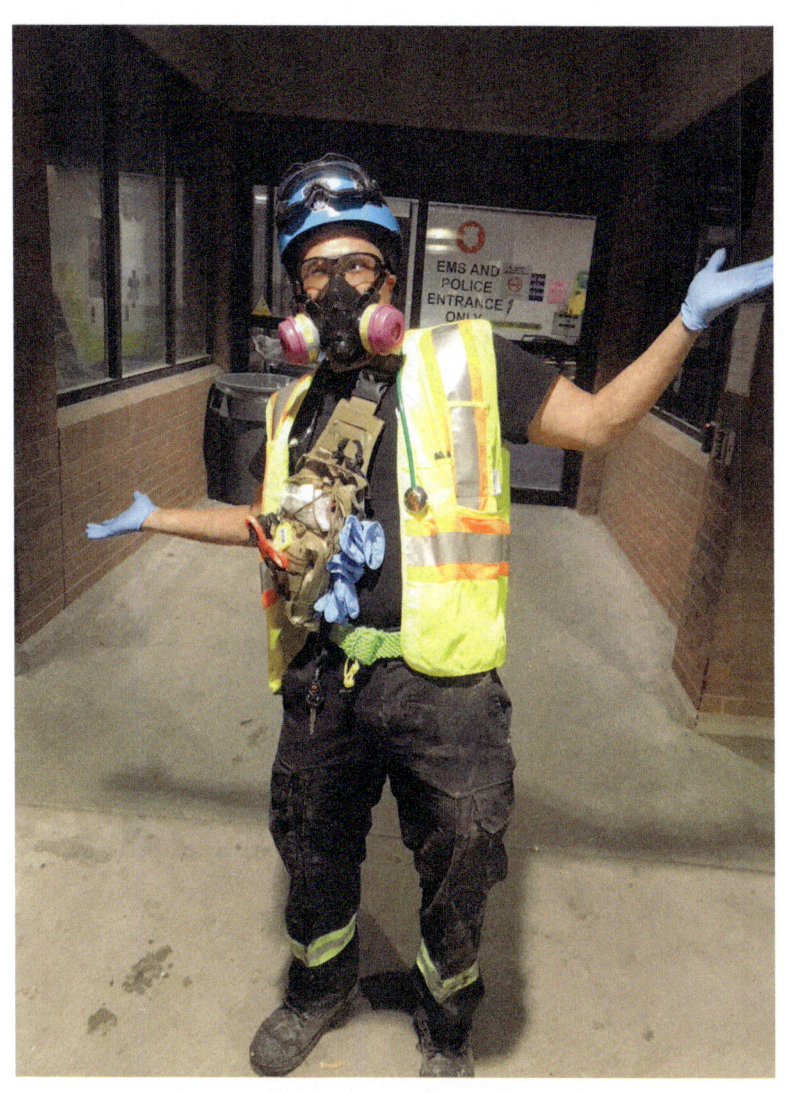

Fresh off of the Niagara Escarpment with my North 7700 respirator at the beginning of the pandemic.

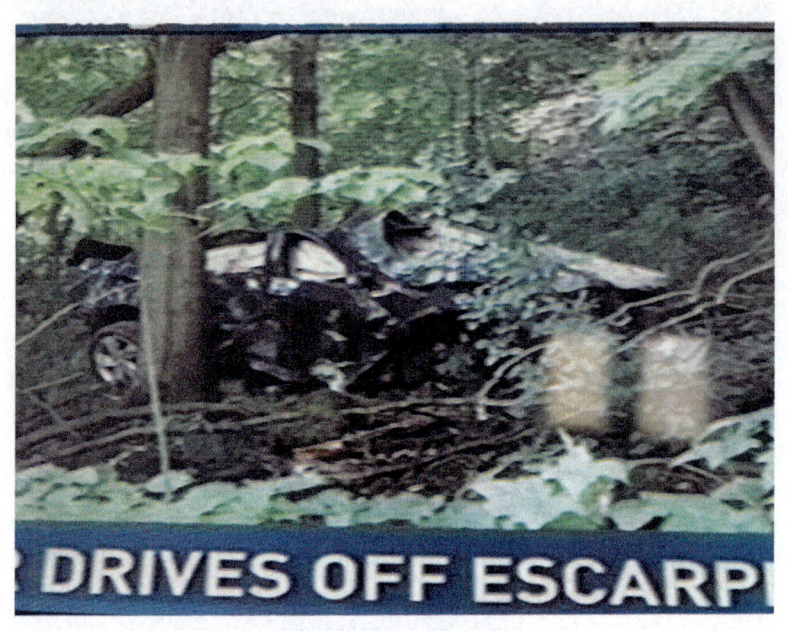

The car that flew off the escarpment.

Chapter 18

Saves

Any paramedic that tells you they don't enjoy saving a life is not telling the truth. Most of us got into the job for it. But a save must meet specific criteria for us. Typically, the patient has to be VSA sometime during the call and then be discharged from the hospital. They must return to the same state they were in before they lost their vital signs. Most of the time, that means walking out of the hospital on their own accord and close to the same mental capacity. Most paramedics wouldn't consider a patient that gets discharged on a home ventilator a true save.

Another example of a save is if you perform a procedure where the patient would have surely died if you didn't. An example would be removing a complete airway obstruction.

There are many times when a patient has no vital signs and we get their heart started again. We call this a return of spontaneous circulation (ROSC). Many of these patients end up on life support in the ICU for some time before they are taken off. I never count those ones as a save. One positive thing that happens in these circumstances is the family gets to gather at the hospital to say goodbye. It provides a closure that is necessary for the grieving process.

My goal when I started as a paramedic was to work thirty years and save a person for each year I worked. Most medics have four or less in their career, so I didn't think this was possible until I looked at my records in 2014 and I had twenty-two. I also noted a massive spike in ROSCs and saves when we changed our focus to early and good quality CPR. Paramedics used to spend too much time reading cardiac rhythms and focusing on skills like IVs and intubation. With the shift to basic and good quality CPR, patient outcomes improved and saves went up.

I cannot take any credit for these saves without acknowledging my partners and allied services that helped me on those calls. Also, these patients received exemplary care at the hospitals that we transported them to. Here are some of my most notable saves.

Season: Fall
Time: 1400hrs
Weather: Cool, clear, 11°c
Area Demographic: Residential house
Dispatch Info: Male in his forties, witnessed collapse

My first save was a man who was forty-one. He had collapsed on the third floor of his home in a sudden cardiac arrest. Being only one year on the job, I was still feeling things out and extremely nervous. I hadn't shocked someone with the defibrillator before, so I was excited to do so. Driving with the lights and sirens on gave me a thrill that has left me in my later years.

I recall coming on-scene and moving quicker than my partner—so quick, I grabbed the defibrillator and ran inside and up the stairs alone, something I don't do anymore. Youth creates haste in retrospect.

"You can't put an old head on new shoulders," one of my best friends said.

Reaching the patient, I only shocked him once and his pulse came back almost immediately.

Hmm, now how are we gonna get him out? I thought.

"Whaddya think? Stair chair, canvas and pole, just a sheet?" I asked my partner.

"He's light, let's just carry him," my partner returned.

So that's what we did. He woke up in the hospital and left against medical advice two days later. I like to think he's still walking around.

Season: Summer
Time: 1230hrs
Weather: Warm, sunny, 23°C
Area Demographic: Urban street corner
Dispatch Info: Self-dispatched

I had a low priority patient in the back and was driving to the hospital when I spotted a small crowd of people gathering at a street corner. One of them jumped out in front of the ambulance, frantically waving his arms, so

I hit the brakes. He pointed to an elderly man that was lying motionless on the ground. I told dispatch to send another unit right away. Dispatch responded that they were already being flooded with calls for this, and backup was on the way.

I went to the back to get the defibrillator from my partner who was with the patient in the ambulance. It would be considered patient abandonment if she left the ambulance to help me, so I was on my own. I moved to the patient, started CPR and got the defibrillator pads on the patient. I shocked him on the curb while onlookers stood in awe.

My supervisor showed up and intubated while I started an IV—my first IV in the field. I couldn't figure out why blood was backing up the line. While my supervisor was tying off the intubation tube, he reached over and pulled off the tourniquet.

This is a classic rookie mistake.

The rest of the call went a little more smoothly. A few shots of epinephrine and a few more shocks got his heart beating again. Although my supervisor laughed off the fact that I forgot to take the tourniquet off, I was pretty displeased with myself. I was young and extremely hard on myself. I had trouble sleeping over these minor mistakes, and it would take years for me to be easier on myself and realize that everything cannot go perfectly on every call.

I had high hopes for a functional recovery for this patient. It was easy to go up to a ward to follow up at this time, so a week later while dropping off a patient at the hospital, I made my way to the ICU. The nurse told me that the patient had gone AWOL from his nursing home that day. The police had put an alert out for him, but he had collapsed on that street corner before the police could find him. She pointed me to his room. I noticed he was tied down to the bed with soft restraints.

"Hey! How are you doing?" I asked.

"I fine!" he said in an accent I couldn't identify.

"Hey uh, why ya tied down?" I asked.

"Nurse say I too much trouble!" he said with a smile.

It was always amazing to see someone's bright personality when the last time you saw them they had none.

Season: Winter
Time: 2230hrs
Weather: Cold, cloudy, 2°C
Area Demographic: Ambulance rendezvous
Dispatch Info: 83yo male, unresponsive, hypotensive

I was at the hospital when I heard a crew call for backup for a patient whose blood pressure dropped and he became unresponsive. I jumped in the ambulance to try and intercept the incoming crew on the road.

We rendezvoused at an intersection a few kilometres from the hospital. The crew updated me that this patient had lived alone and missed a week of dialysis. This usually yields a condition called hyperkalemia, or too much potassium. These patients are prone to sudden cardiac arrest. I got a line and tried to get his blood pressure up with fluid. Just outside the hospital, his heart went into a lethal arrhythmia and I lost his pulse. I shocked him only once and he regained his pulse.

We made haste to the ER and transferred care over to the emergency doc. The hospital treated him for hyperkalemia and told us his prognosis was poor because of his age. He wouldn't come off life support.

Even though statistics were against his outcome, I still thought he had a slight chance at recovery, so I went up to the ICU the following week. I looked at what I thought was my patient on life support. I talked to the nurse, and she told me he was not the hyperkalemic patient. She pointed to the room next door where my patient was sitting up in a chair eating soup and watching television. I smiled and went to grab a coffee for my partner.

Season: Winter
Time: 1100hrs
Weather: Cool, 5°C
Area Demographic: Karate dojo
Dispatch Info: Chest pain

I heard the address go out and knew it was my old friend's karate dojo. Dispatch gave the call to another ambulance, but I knew we were closer by at least half the distance, so I volunteered.

I hadn't seen my buddy Tyler in more than a few years. We fought together on a junior team travelling the United States in the mid-nineties. I went to drive an ambulance and he started a karate school. I think he now owns four of them and they are franchised.

"STEVE!" Tyler shouted, hands in the air.

"Buddy!" I shouted as we briefly shook hands.

Our reunion was mere seconds as Tyler directed my attention to a man in his mid-forties sitting on a bench. He was sweating, pale and looked like he was going to throw up. Tyler introduced me to his student, and I got a bad feeling about it right away, so I got him on my stretcher. Tyler told me that the student was just getting back from a few months' hiatus and they were performing self-defence moves for a routine—not even doing them to full capacity. That is when he got nauseated and complained of chest pain. Tyler was really concerned that the pain travelled down his left arm. I realized there had been a class going on and there were about twenty onlookers. Now on my stretcher, he was lying down and said he didn't feel right.

I have a bad feeling about this, my mind repeated.

No sooner did I think this then he went into a full-blown seizure, the kind you have before your heart stops. Right in front of my friend and his karate school. I felt his neck for a pulse and there was none. My partner was on the radio and already asking for the fire department—we would need extra hands for this one. I quickly cut his belt (green belt with a black strip)—a blasphemy in the karate world, but it was necessary for speed. If my hunch was right, we needed to shock this guy ASAP to get his heart started again. As fast as my partner and I could move, we got the pads on, charged up the defibrillator and whacked this guy with 120 joules of electricity.

I watched the cardiac monitor and saw an ECG with a pulse. I confirmed this with a pulse check at his neck. *Whew!* In a few moments, he woke up and made us look like we knew what we were doing. At that moment the fire department arrived.

"What happened?" the patient asked.

Linda, a firefighter I knew well said, "Hey Stevie! I thought he was vital signs absent?"

What timing they had.

Stunned, I replied, "Uhhhh, he was, but now he's not."

That was all I could come up with.

"What does that mean? What just happened?" the patient said with increased concern in his voice.

"Listen, your heart stopped, but we got it started again," I said.

"Can I call my wife?" he asked.

"Not right at this moment," I said.

I had so many things to get done in the short transport time. In my haste, I forgot to let him make the call and still feel guilty about it to this day. This happened when I was pretty seasoned but still a little excitable. Nowadays I might be able to remember something like that in a critical call. Again, it's me being hard on myself. I got him to the hospital alive.

James gave me a framed ECG of the single shock that saved that man's life—he always gave me thoughtful gifts like that. Eventually, the patient found me on Facebook, and his profile pic had him wearing a shirt that said, "I survived the widowmaker" His name was Colin. Talking with James, we decided that Colin would very much appreciate the ECG as a gift. I dropped it off at the karate school along with a green belt with a black stripe. One karateka to another. He later got that ECG tattooed on his inner forearm.

Season: Spring
Time: 1800hrs
Weather: BBQ worthy
Area Demographic: Urban core
Dispatch Info: Man choking

The call came in just as we started our night shift. Dispatch told us it was right around the corner. From the time the call came in to the time we were on-scene was only four minutes. There was a family BBQ going on as we were led to the backyard. The smell of smoked sausage filled my nose. There was a bystander doing compressions on the patient, and I encouraged him to keep going as I approached the patient. One of the firefighters pointed out that the patient was on a closed hot tub cover—not an ideal surface for resuscitation. I thanked him and we promptly moved him to the grass.

The patient was a forty-year-old male, 250 pounds. His face was completely purple and his mouth was moving but he was not breathing. My partner got the monitor on while I worked on his airway.

"What was he eating?" I asked.

"Hot dog and coleslaw!" someone replied.

I had the patient on his side and was finger sweeping his airway while my partner got the suction out. I now knew what the white, creamy, leafy substance coming out of his mouth was. The suction was ready, and I started using it in his airway.

"Heart rate 170, spo2 70, Steve," James called out to me.

Both told me he was very close to death if I didn't get his airway cleared within the next few moments.

My partner was getting the intubation kit open as I started to use the portable suction machine. After suctioning out white goopy coleslaw, I heard the suction motor rev to its max, which indicates that there is something stuck to the end of it. A piece of hot dog that is four centimetres square came out, must have been a jumbo! The man instantly started breathing again. I listened carefully and observed that there seemed to be no more airway obstruction. He began to vomit, and I encouraged him to keep it up. After a few minutes, he sat up and everyone could finally breathe a sigh of relief.

We gathered some medical info and found out that he'd had a traumatic brain injury before and had trouble swallowing sometimes. Because of how close this man was to death, we rolled lights and sirens to the hospital.

We arrived at the hospital without incident, and the man was set to make a full recovery. Over a coffee, my partner and I discussed how all the stars must have been aligned. So many things contributed to his outcome. Our base was close. We got to him quickly. Removed the obstruction promptly, had good teamwork, etc. James and I recognized that this call was a save. I nodded and smiled—my thirtieth save. After seventeen years and 310 vital signs absent patients, I had achieved my goal. I asked my partner to take a picture back at base.

Later during paramedic week, I asked permission from my chief to post my achievement on Facebook. I even got on the local news during that week. I wouldn't stop there, of course. To the end of my paramedic days, I'll try and continue the trend.

As the years passed, patient confidentiality became more secure and following up on a patient was more difficult. The pandemic made it almost impossible for that to happen. Initially it upset me that I couldn't find out if a patient had walked away from a cardiac arrest, but I had matured as a person and was much older than when I had set the goal over twenty years before. It has become more important for me to let go of recording a save, in favour of focussing on good patient care. The by-product of that will produce the best chance of any patient's survival.

Chapter song selection:
"Walking on Sunshine" by Katrina and the Waves

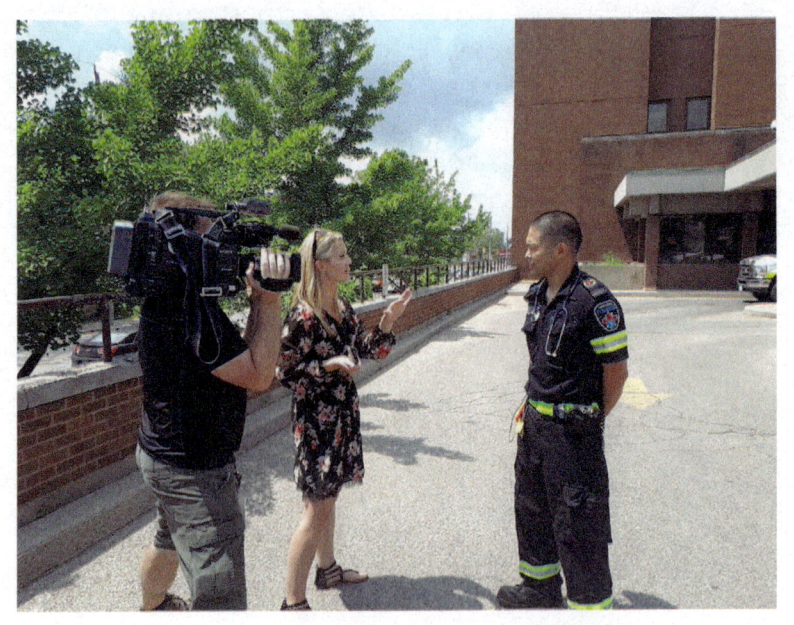

I got a small segment on the news during paramedic week for my thirty saves.

EPILOGUE

Thanks for coming along for a ride in the ambulance with me. I hope you found my stories interesting, informative and emotional. It's been a roller coaster of a journey in the past twenty-plus years. With any luck, I'll retire at fifty-five.

Moving slower with a few more wrinkles on my face will be a badge I've earned. Recovering from a string of busy night shifts won't be any easier. But in the end, I'll leave this job with a sense of duty and completion.

The next time you see an ambulance in your rear-view mirror with lights and sirens, pull over and stop for us. You never know what kind of emergency we are going to or coming from. Thanks again for reading.

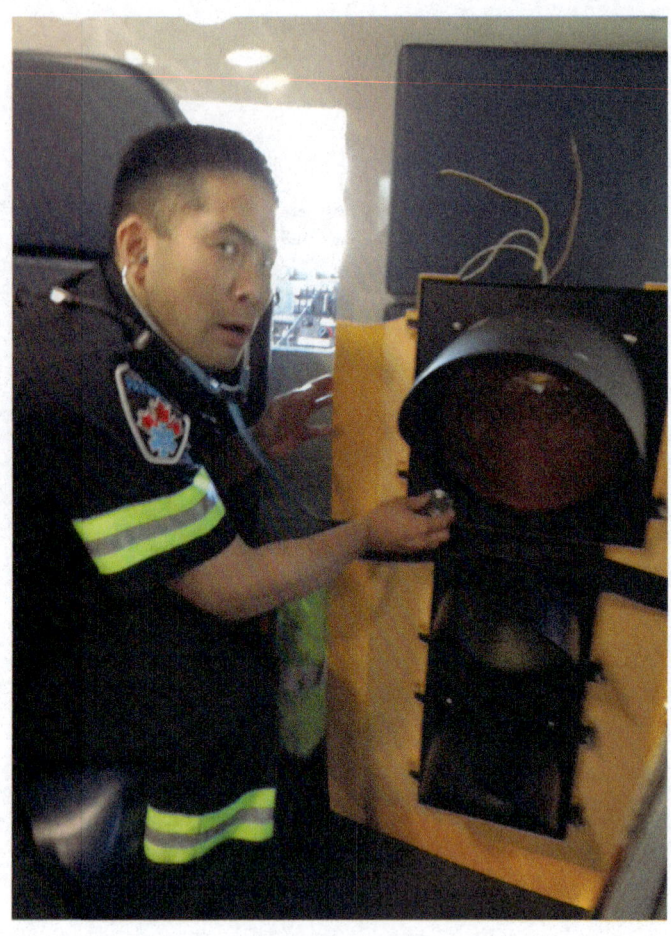

No heart sounds! During an extremely windy day my partner and I witnessed this traffic light fall into the middle of the intersection. James and I picked it up for safety reasons and dropped it off a nearby hospital where city employees could pick it up. Having fun at work is also an essential paramedic survival tool.

Printed in Great Britain
by Amazon